Department of Veterans Affairs
Health Services Research & Development Service | Evidence-based Synthesis Program

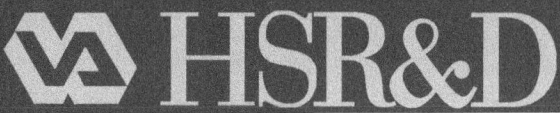 

I0470824

Delirium: Screening, Prevention, and Diagnosis – A Systematic Review of the Evidence

September 2011

Prepared for:

Department of Veterans Affairs
Veterans Health Administration
Health Services Research & Development Service
Washington, DC 20420

Prepared by:

Evidence-based Synthesis Program (ESP) Center
Minneapolis VA Medical Center
Minneapolis, MN
Timothy J. Wilt, MD, MPH, Director

Investigators:

Principal Investigator:
Rebecca Rossom, MD, MSCR

Co-Investigators:
Pauline Anderson, RN
Nancy Greer, PhD

Research Associates:
Roderick MacDonald, MS
Indulis Rutks, BS
James Tacklind, BS

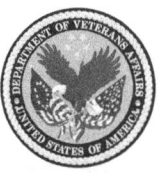

PREFACE

Health Services Research & Development Service's (HSR&D's) Evidence-based Synthesis Program (ESP) was established to provide timely and accurate syntheses of targeted healthcare topics of particular importance to Veterans Affairs (VA) managers and policymakers, as they work to improve the health and healthcare of Veterans. The ESP disseminates these reports throughout VA.

HSR&D provides funding for four ESP Centers and each Center has an active VA affiliation. The ESP Centers generate evidence syntheses on important clinical practice topics, and these reports help:

- develop clinical policies informed by evidence,
- guide the implementation of effective services to improve patient outcomes and to support VA clinical practice guidelines and performance measures, and
- set the direction for future research to address gaps in clinical knowledge.

In 2009, the ESP Coordinating Center was created to expand the capacity of HSR&D Central Office and the four ESP sites by developing and maintaining program processes. In addition, the Center established a Steering Committee comprised of HSR&D field-based investigators, VA Patient Care Services, Office of Quality and Performance, and Veterans Integrated Service Networks (VISN) Clinical Management Officers. The Steering Committee provides program oversight, guides strategic planning, coordinates dissemination activities, and develops collaborations with VA leadership to identify new ESP topics of importance to Veterans and the VA healthcare system.

Comments on this evidence report are welcome and can be sent to Nicole Floyd, ESP Coordinating Center Program Manager, at nicole.floyd@va.gov.

Recommended citation: Greer N, Rossom R, Anderson P, MacDonald R, Tacklind J, Rutks I, Wilt TJ. Delirium: Screening, Prevention, and Diagnosis - A Systematic Review of the Evidence. VA-ESP Project #09-009; 2011.

This report is based on research conducted by the Evidence-based Synthesis Program (ESP) Center located at the Minneapolis VA Medical Center, Minneapolis, MN funded by the Department of Veterans Affairs, Veterans Health Administration, Office of Research and Development, Health Services Research and Development. The findings and conclusions in this document are those of the author(s) who are responsible for its contents; the findings and conclusions do not necessarily represent the views of the Department of Veterans Affairs or the United States government. Therefore, no statement in this article should be construed as an official position of the Department of Veterans Affairs. No investigators have any affiliations or financial involvement (e.g., employment, consultancies, honoraria, stock ownership or options, expert testimony, grants or patents received or pending, or royalties) that conflict with material presented in the report.

TABLE OF CONTENTS

TABLES

FIGURES

APPENDIX A. SEARCH STRATEGIES

APPENDIX B. STUDY SELECTION FORM

APPENDIX C. PEER REVIEW COMMENTS/AUTHOR RESPONSES

APPENDIX D. EVIDENCE TABLES

EXECUTIVE SUMMARY

BACKGROUND

Delirium is a common syndrome in hospitalized or institutionalized adults. It is characterized by the acute onset of altered mental status, hallmarked by difficulty sustaining attention and a fluctuating course. Delirium frequently causes patients, families, and health care providers considerable distress. The incidence varies widely based on patient population, setting, and intensity of diagnostic ascertainment with reported values of 10% to over 80%. Delirium is associated with multiple serious outcomes including increased morbidity, length of hospital stay, healthcare costs, institutionalization, and mortality.[1,2,3] In surgical settings, older adults and those with multiple medical conditions are at increased risk for postoperative delirium.[4] Delirium may be under-recognized by healthcare providers and it can be difficult to resolve.[5,6] Several brief "bedside" questionnaires and checklists exist that can help detect delirium earlier and among those with milder symptoms. Additionally, efforts to prevent the development of delirium in those at risk have been advocated.[3,6] Medications (including sedatives, narcotics, and anticholinergic drugs), diseases and intercurrent illnesses (e.g., stroke, infection, shock, anemia), surgical procedures (especially orthopedic and cardiac surgery), and environmental factors (e.g., use of a bladder catheter, pain, and emotional stress) are all associated with delirium.[3,7] Therefore, identifying and implementing effective strategies to prevent and detect delirium could improve clinical outcomes and resource utilization. Suggested strategies to prevent delirium include avoidance of psychoactive medications, pharmacologic interventions to decrease risk, and single- or multi-component non-pharmacologic interventions (including use of music, mobilization, fluid and nutrition management, and orientation and cognitive stimulation).[4,6,7]

This review was undertaken to evaluate the effectiveness of screening for delirium, the effectiveness and harms of strategies to prevent delirium, and the comparative diagnostic accuracy of tools used to detect delirium. Specifically, we addressed the following key questions:

1.   What is the *effectiveness* of *screening* for delirium in adult inpatients?
     a. Do these results vary by medical unit, age, gender or comorbid conditions?
     b. Does screening for delirium improve clinical outcomes?
2.   What are the *effectiveness and harms* of delirium *prevention* strategies in acute elderly inpatients?
     a. Do these results vary by medical unit, age, gender or comorbid conditions?
3.   What is the comparative *diagnostic accuracy* of the tools used to detect delirium:
     a. In elderly medical and surgical inpatients?
     b. In elderly medical or surgical intensive care unit (ICU) inpatients?

METHODS

We searched MEDLINE, CINAHL, and PsycINFO from 1950 to November 2010 using standard search terms (Appendix A). We limited the search to peer-reviewed articles involving human subjects and published in the English language. Additional citations were identified from reference lists and Technical Expert Panel members. Titles and abstracts were reviewed by physicians, nurses, and research assistants trained in the critical analysis of literature. Full text versions of potentially relevant articles were similarly reviewed. Study characteristics, patient characteristics, and outcomes were extracted and evidence and outcomes tables, organized by key question, were created under the supervision of the Principal Investigator, a geriatric psychiatrist.

We assessed study quality of randomized trials of prevention strategies (Key Question 2) according to the following criteria: 1) adequate allocation concealment, 2) blinding of key study personnel, 3) analysis by intention-to-treat, and 4) reporting of number of withdrawals/dropouts by group assignment. Study quality of studies reported for Key Question 3 (studies of diagnostic accuracy) was assessed using the method described in the Rationale Clinical Examination series.[8]

DATA SYNTHESIS

We constructed evidence tables showing the study characteristics and results for all included studies. We critically analyzed studies to compare their characteristics, methods, and findings. Pooled analyses were performed, where feasible, for studies of prevention strategies. All other data were narratively summarized.

PEER REVIEW

A draft version of this report was reviewed by technical experts, as well as VA clinical leadership. Reviewer comments were addressed and our responses incorporated in the final report.

RESULTS

For the screening question, we identified 1,889 abstracts and excluded 1,778. We reviewed the full text of 111 references and none met inclusion criteria. For prevention, we identified 1,175 abstracts and excluded 947. Of 228 full text articles reviewed, 31 met eligibility criteria. We added 8 references from hand-searching for a total of 39 included references. For diagnostic accuracy in intensive care units, we identified 76 abstracts and excluded 40 of those. Of 36 full text articles reviewed, 15 met inclusion criteria.

KEY QUESTION #1. What is the effectiveness of screening for delirium in adult inpatients?
1a. Do these results vary by medical unit, age, gender or comorbid conditions?
1b. Does screening for delirium improve clinical outcomes?

We identified no randomized controlled trials of screening for delirium in hospitalized patients. There is no direct evidence that screening for delirium is beneficial or harmful. However, while potentially beneficial, universal screening may also pose harms, such as misclassification, subsequent treatment of non-delirious patients, or failure to accurately identify or intervene on delirious patients. Additionally, we found no evidence from recent systematic reviews that pharmacologic and non-pharmacologic treatments improve outcomes for patients with screen-detected delirium. Therefore, we conclude that the evidence is insufficient about the net benefit of delirium screening among all hospitalized patients or subgroups of patients as defined by age, gender, comorbidities or admission to intensive care units.

KEY QUESTION #2. What are the effectiveness and harms of delirium prevention strategies in acute elderly inpatients?
2a. Do these results vary by medical unit, age, gender or comorbid conditions?

We identified randomized and non-randomized trials of pharmacologic and non-pharmacologic strategies for prevention of delirium. Studies using pharmacologic interventions to prevent delirium were few in number, small in size, and examined different categories of prevention medications often in unique patient populations and settings. Moderate level evidence from two studies of atypical antipsychotics and low level evidence from one study each of analgesia via fascia iliaca compartmental block (pre- and post-operative), lighter anesthesia, or post-operative sedation with dexmedetomidine suggests that these pharmacological approaches may reduce the incidence of delirium following orthopedic or cardiac surgery. There was no difference in delirium incidence associated with the use of cholinesterase inhibitors, statins, a benzodiazepine/opioid protocol, or regional versus general anesthesia and the evidence for using typical antipsychotics is mixed. Multi-component strategies varied greatly but often included staff education plus additional components such as geriatric consultation, individual care planning, focused prevention of infection, improving mobility, frequent orientation, bowel and bladder care regimens, insomnia protocols, adequate pain management, minimizing psychoactive or sedating medications, and maintaining adequate hydration and nutrition. Strategies were generally successful in preventing delirium but intervention variability and lack of assessment of individual intervention components made it difficult to determine which components may be effective. Limited evidence suggests that staff education alone or music therapy may be effective strategies. In one small study, bright light therapy was found to be not effective for delirium prevention. Harms were infrequent and mild.

None of the included studies were stratified by medical unit, age, gender, or comorbid conditions although two studies enrolled only men. There is insufficient evidence to determine whether the effects of different preventive strategies vary by medical unit, age, gender, or comorbid conditions.

KEY QUESTION #3. What is the comparative diagnostic accuracy of the tools used to detect delirium:
3a. In elderly medical and surgical inpatients?
3b. In elderly ICU inpatients?

A systematic review of the comparative effectiveness of bedside instruments concluded that the Confusion Assessment Method (CAM) was a suitable tool for medical and surgical inpatients, many of whom were evaluated in geriatric units. Using Diagnostic and Statistical Manual of

Mental Disorders (DSM) criteria performed by a specialist physician as a reference standard, the pooled sensitivity and specificity of the CAM were 86% and 93%, respectively. The pooled likelihood ratio for a positive test was 9.6 (95%CI 5.8 to 16.0). The pooled likelihood ratio for a negative test was 0.16 (95%CI 0.09 to 0.29). However, there was considerable heterogeneity in the 12 studies. The ease of administration (completion in less than 5 minutes) was also considered although it was noted that administrators should be trained for optimal use and that the CAM was originally developed for use in conjunction with a formal cognitive assessment. The accuracy of bedside instruments delivered by individuals without training as stand-alone tools for delirium screening is not known.

Fewer studies have evaluated the diagnostic accuracy of tools to detect delirium for elderly intensive care unit (ICU) inpatients. The CAM-ICU, a version of the CAM adapted for use in the ICU, appears to have high specificity but the sensitivity is less consistent (ranging from 64 to 100%) indicating that some patients with delirium will not be identified using the CAM-ICU alone. Other tools have been evaluated in only one or two studies.

FUTURE RESEARCH

The highest future research need is to conduct a large multicenter pragmatic randomized trial to evaluate the clinical effectiveness and harms of screening for delirium in a broad spectrum of patients admitted to hospitals. More research is needed to verify the findings that pharmacologic and non-pharmacologic strategies can prevent delirium, particularly in larger and more diverse populations, and with reports stratified by age, medical unit, and comorbid conditions. Additionally, more research is needed to identify which components of the multi-component non-pharmacologic strategies may be most successful in delirium prevention. Finally, continued evaluation of diagnostic tools (especially bed side tools in stand-alone settings administered by clinical personnel) is warranted especially across a wide range of populations and settings.

EVIDENCE REPORT

INTRODUCTION

This review was undertaken to evaluate the effectiveness of screening for delirium in adult inpatients, the effectiveness of strategies employed to prevent delirium in acute elderly inpatients, and the comparative diagnostic accuracy of tools used to detect delirium in elderly medical, surgical, and ICU patients.

For this review, we were careful to make the important distinction between screening for delirium (testing all patients for delirium without a prior index of suspicion) and diagnosis of delirium (testing those patients for whom there is already some suspicion of delirium).

BACKGROUND

Delirium is a common syndrome, characterized by the acute onset of altered mental status, hallmarked by difficulty sustaining attention and a fluctuating course, and frequently causing patients, families, and health care providers considerable distress. There have been wide variations in the reported incidence of delirium in medical inpatients, largely due to differences in setting, patient population, and methodology. It has been estimated that 10-30% of patients admitted to the hospital develop delirium;[9,10] this percentage can increase significantly in at-risk populations, including frail elderly patients (estimated at 60%),[11] post-surgical elderly patients (estimated as high as 89%),[12] or ICU patients (estimated at 41%).[13]

Delirium has been associated with multiple serious outcomes in medically ill patients, including increased morbidity, length of stay, healthcare costs, institutionalization, and mortality.[2,3,14-16] Delirium is often significantly under-recognized by healthcare providers and can frequently be difficult to resolve.[5,6,17,18] Several brief "bedside" questionnaires and checklists exist that can detect delirium earlier and among those with milder symptoms. Efforts to prevent the development of delirium in those at risk have been advocated.[3,6] Medications (including sedatives, narcotics, and anticholinergic drugs), diseases and intercurrent illnesses (e.g., stroke, infection, shock, anemia), surgical procedures (especially orthopedic and cardiac surgery), and environmental factors (e.g., use of a bladder catheter, pain, and emotional stress) are all precipitating factors for delirium development.[6,7] Therefore, identifying and implementing effective strategies to prevent and detect delirium could improve clinical outcomes and resource utilization. Suggested strategies to prevent delirium include avoidance of psychoactive medications, pharmacologic interventions to decrease risk, and single- or multi-component non-pharmacologic interventions (including use of music, mobilization, fluid and nutrition management, and orientation and cognitive stimulation).[4,6,7]

METHODS

TOPIC DEVELOPMENT

This project was nominated by Nancy Schmid, ADPNS, a Nurse Executive at Syracuse VA Medical Center, with input from a technical expert panel of clinicians, researchers, and administrators.

The final key questions are:

1. What is the *effectiveness* of *screening* for delirium in adult inpatients?
    a. Do these results vary by medical unit, age, gender or comorbid conditions?
    b. Does screening for delirium improve clinical outcomes?
2. What are the *effectiveness and harms* of delirium *prevention* strategies in acute elderly inpatients?
    a. Do these results vary by medical unit, age, gender or comorbid conditions?
3. What is the comparative *diagnostic accuracy* of the tools used to detect   delirium:
    a. In elderly medical and surgical inpatients?
    b. In elderly medical or surgical intensive care unit (ICU) inpatients?

An analytic framework (Figure 1) was developed to depict the potential pathway of a hospitalized adult patient. This report will focus on the outcomes and harms associated with screening (Key Question #1), preventive interventions (Key Questions #2), and diagnosis (Key Question #3).

Figure 1. Analytic Framework

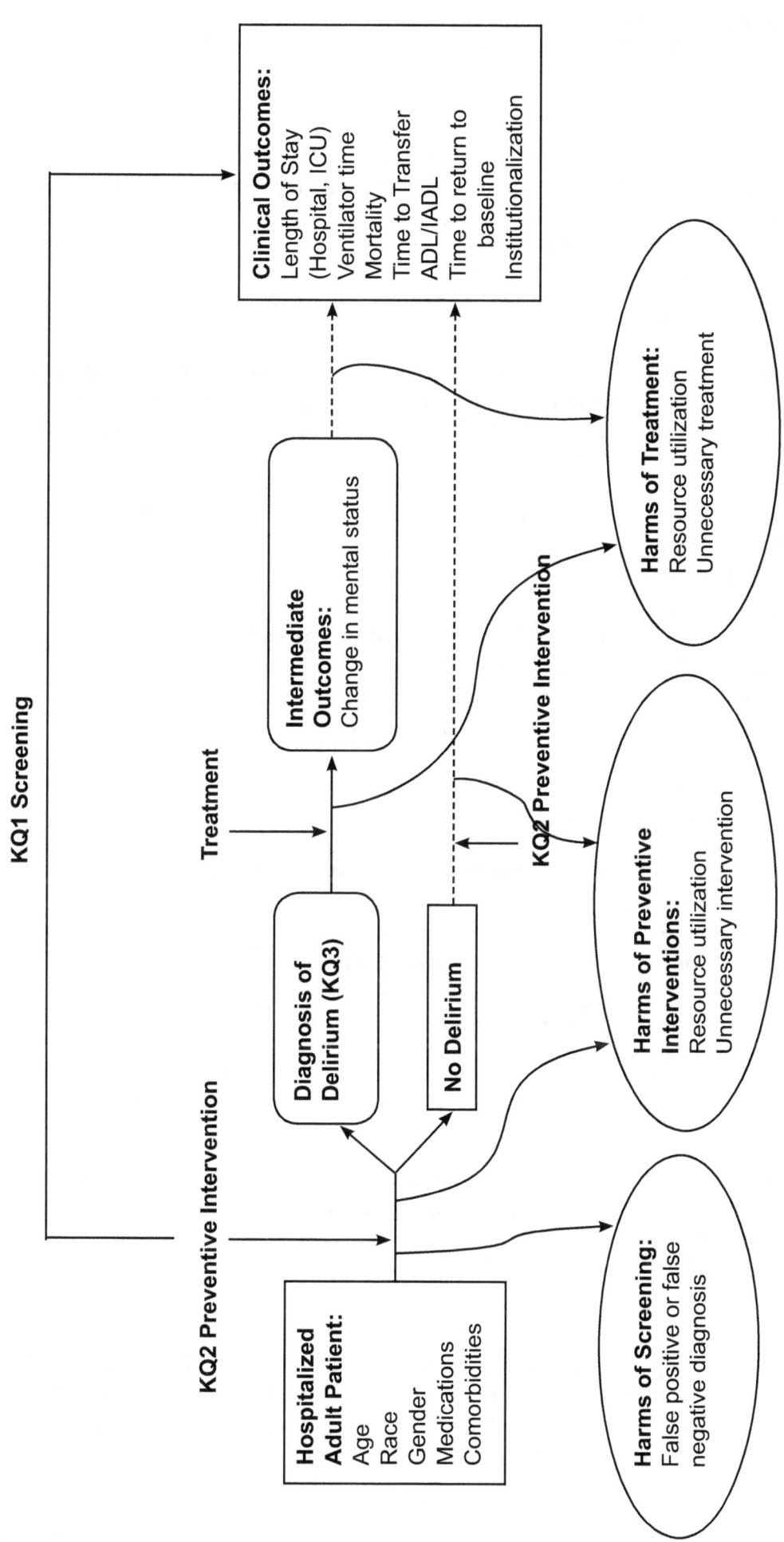

SEARCH STRATEGY

We searched MEDLINE, CINAHL, and PsycINFO from 1950 to November 2010 using standard search terms (Appendix A). We limited the search to peer-reviewed articles involving human subjects and published in the English language. Additional citations were identified from reference lists and Technical Expert Panel members.

STUDY SELECTION

Physicians, nurses, and research assistants trained in the critical analysis of literature assessed for relevance the abstracts of citations identified from literature searches. Full-text articles of potentially relevant abstracts were retrieved for further review. A Study Selection Form (Appendix B) was used to guide this review.

Specific exclusion criteria for the screening and diagnosis questions were as follows:
1) Non-English publication
2) Population <16 yrs old
3) Alcohol-related delirium
4) Not hospitalized patients (nursing home or similar was excluded)
5) No reference standard (DSM III, III-R, or IV)
6) Index test and reference standard performed by same individual
7) Case series (<10 patients), case report, editorial, letter
8) Not patients with delirium
9) No outcomes of interest
10) Not a screening or diagnosis study

Specific exclusion criteria for the prevention question were as follows:
1) Non-English publication
2) Population <16 years old
3) Nursing home residents (or mixed hospital/nursing home if unable to get results of hospital only)
4) Case series, case report, editorial, letter
5) Not about delirium prevention

DATA ABSTRACTION

Study characteristics, patient characteristics, and outcomes were extracted and evidence and outcomes tables, organized by key question, were created under the supervision of the Principal Investigator, a geriatric psychiatrist.

QUALITY ASSESSMENT

We assessed study quality of randomized trials of prevention strategies (Key Question 2) according to the following criteria: 1) adequate allocation concealment, 2) blinding of key study personnel, 3) analysis by intention-to-treat, and 4) reporting of number of withdrawals/dropouts by group assignment.[19] Studies were rated as good, fair, or poor quality. A rating of good generally indicated that the trial reported adequate allocation concealment, blinding, analysis by intent-to-treat, and reasons for dropouts/attrition were reported. Studies were generally rated poor if the method of allocation concealment was inadequate or not defined, blinding was not defined, analysis by intent-to-treat was not utilized, and reasons for dropouts/attrition were not reported and/or there was a high rate of attrition.

Study quality of studies reported for Key Question 3 (studies of diagnostic accuracy) was assessed using the method described in the Rationale Clinical Examination series.[8] Briefly, studies are designated as Level of Evidence 1 if they present an independent, blinded comparison with a criterion standard in a large number (defined as 100 or more patients in the delirium diagnosis review) of consecutive individuals suspected of having the target condition or a Level of Evidence 2 if they meet all the criteria for Level 1 but enroll fewer than 100 patients. Level of Evidence 3 studies are similar to Level 1 or Level 2 studies but do not enroll patients consecutively. Studies with a non-independent comparison with the criterion standard and that enroll (at least in part) patients who obviously have the target condition are designated as Level of Evidence 4. Studies with a reference test of questionable validity are designated Level of Evidence 5.

DATA SYNTHESIS

We constructed evidence tables showing the study characteristics and results for all included studies, organized by key question. We critically analyzed studies to compare their characteristics, methods, and findings. Pooled analyses were performed, where feasible, for studies of prevention strategies. All other data were narratively summarized.

RATING THE BODY OF EVIDENCE

We assessed the overall quality of evidence for randomized trials of prevention strategies (Key Question #2) using the method reported by Owens et al.[20] Briefly, for each outcome evaluated, the strength of the evidence was assessed based on: (1) risk of bias; (2) consistency; (3) directness; and (4) precision. Based on these four domains, the overall evidence was rated as: (1) high, meaning high confidence that the evidence reflects the true effect; (2) moderate, indicating moderate confidence that further research may change our confidence in the estimate of effect and may change the estimate; (3) low, meaning there is low confidence that the evidence reflects the true effect; and (4) insufficient, indicating that evidence either is unavailable or does not permit a conclusion. Due to heterogeneity in the interventions evaluated, we did not rate the overall strength of evidence for the non-randomized trials.

PEER REVIEW

A draft version of this report was reviewed by technical experts and VA clinical leadership. Their comments and our responses are presented in Appendix C.

RESULTS

LITERATURE FLOW

For the screening question, we identified 1,889 abstracts and excluded 1,778. We reviewed the full text of 111 references and none met inclusion criteria.

For the prevention question, we identified 1,175 abstract and excluded 947. Of 228 full text articles reviewed, 31 met eligibility criteria. We added 8 references from hand-searching for a total of 39 included references. In addition to our literature search, we identified one recent Cochrane systematic review of delirium prevention[21] and a recent National Institute for Health and Clinical Excellence (NICE) guideline on diagnosis, prevention, and management of delirium.[7,22] Five of the six randomized controlled trials included in the Cochrane review are included in our analysis. The sixth trial, a study of prophylactic citicoline (a psychostimulant) versus placebo, was published in Spanish language and was therefore not eligible for our review. The authors reported no difference in delirium incidence.[23]

The NICE guideline cited seven studies of pharmacologic prevention strategies, five studies of non-pharmacologic strategies, and eight studies of multi-component interventions. Six of the pharmacologic studies, one of the non-pharmacologic studies, and seven of the multi-component studies met our inclusion criteria and are included in our analysis. The remaining studies were either not conducted in a hospital setting or did not provide data on outcomes of interest.

For the question about diagnostic accuracy, our search was limited to studies of patients admitted to intensive care units. We identified 76 abstracts and excluded 40 of those. Of 36 full text articles reviewed, 15 met inclusion criteria. Figures 2, 3, and 4 present the literature search results.

Figure 2. Flow Diagram – Delirium Screening Studies

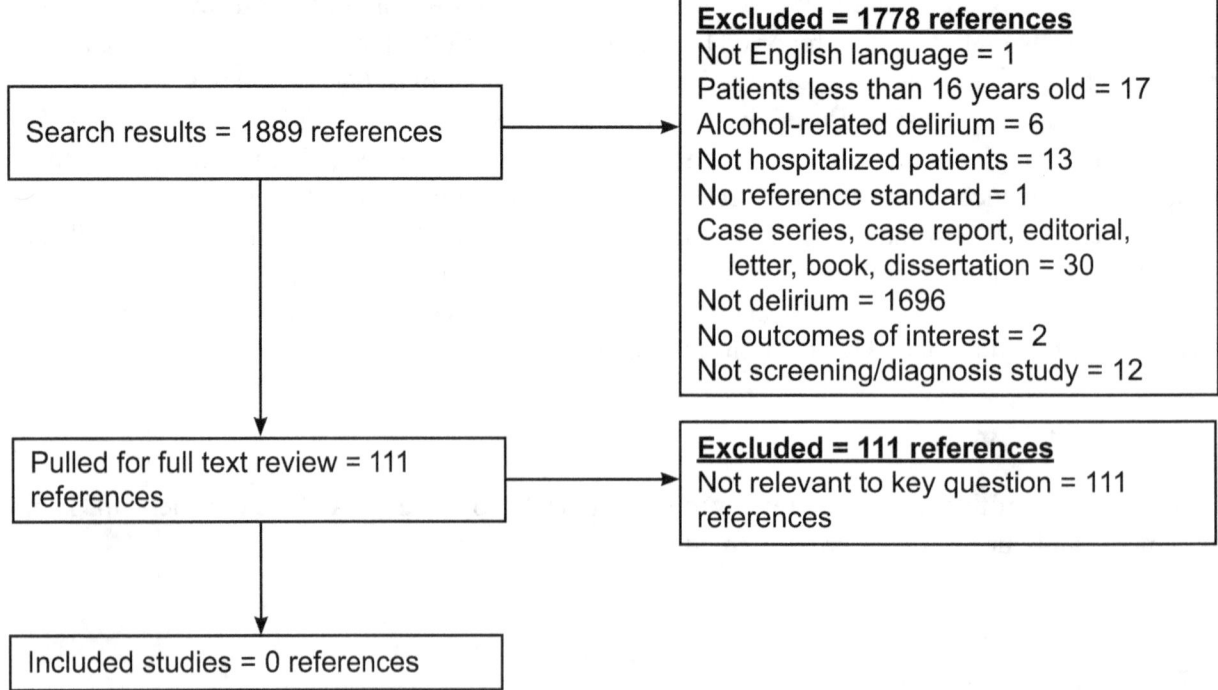

Figure 3. Flow Diagram – Delirium Prevention Studies

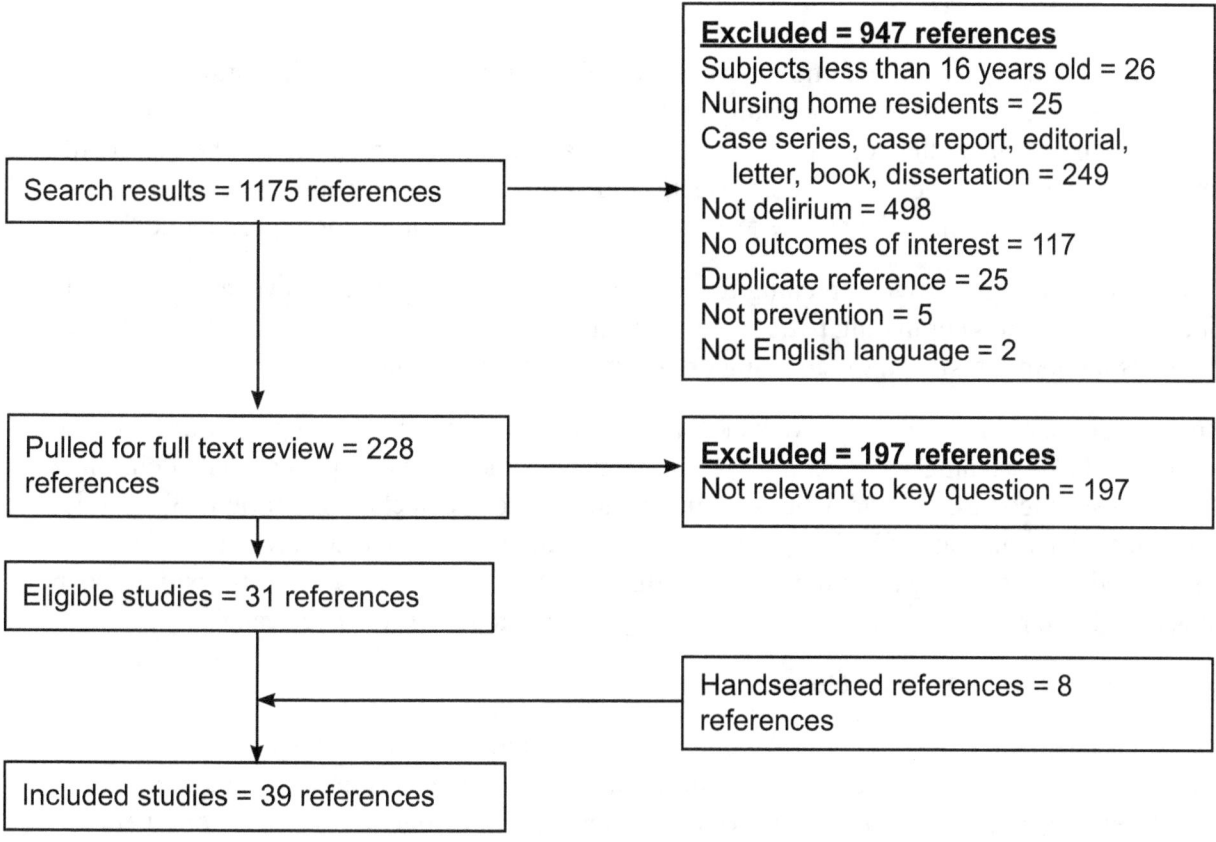

Figure 4. Flow Diagram – Delirium ICU Diagnosis Studies

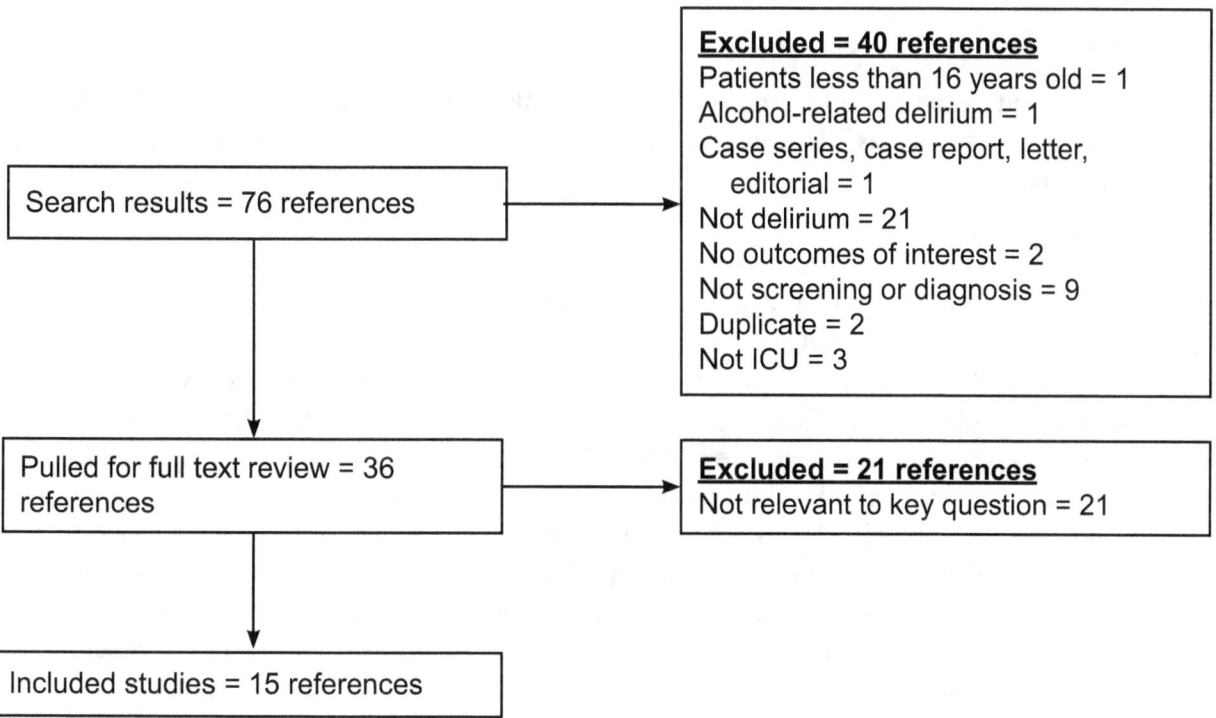

KEY QUESTION #1. What is the effectiveness of screening for delirium in adult inpatients?

Screening for a disease or condition is warranted if the disease is serious, if treatment before symptoms are evident reduces morbidity and mortality, and if the prevalence of preclinical disease is high among the population screened.[24] In addition, the screening test should identify most or all with the condition, be cost effective and ethical, be easy to administer, and impose minimal discomfort on patients. The test must also be reliable, valid, and reproducible.[25]

Based on the criteria above, screening for delirium may be appropriate. However, we did not identify any studies comparing patient outcomes in hospitalized (including intensive care unit) patients randomly assigned to screening or no screening for delirium.

In the absence of direct evidence we look for indirect links between screening and outcomes. To indirectly link screening and outcomes, we would need evidence that 1) patients with delirium have worse outcomes, 2) systematic screening would improve detection of delirium, 3) treatments for detected delirium are effective, particularly if delirium can be detected early, and 4) harms associated with screening are minimal. A systematic review for this evidence is beyond the scope of this report. We report results from recent existing systematic reviews where available.

Outcomes in Patients with Delirium

A 2006 systematic review reported outcomes from 19 study cohorts.[26] Study design, diagnostic method, patient selection criteria, comorbid conditions, length of follow-up, outcome measurement, and adjustment (or lack of adjustment) for potential confounders varied among the studies making conclusions difficult. Overall, there appeared to be increased mortality in patients with delirium. Results for hospital length of stay, resolution of symptoms at discharge, institutionalization at discharge, and functional ability at discharge were less consistent.

Improved Detection

If all hospitalized patients or all patients at increased risk were screened for delirium, detection would be expected to increase. However, we did not identify any systematic reviews on detection rates with screening.

Treatment

A search of the literature identified several recent systematic reviews that focused on treatment. A 2007 Cochrane review included data from 3 randomized trials that compared antipsychotic medications used to treat delirium.[27] No differences in patient outcomes or adverse events were found between low-dose haloperidol, risperidone, and olanzapine. A second review included 14 studies, 9 single-agent and 5 comparative.[28] None of the studies included a placebo control group and the total sample size was 448. Although most subjects experienced improvements in delirium severity, without a blinded placebo comparison group it is impossible to determine the role of the study medication in the observed improvement. Few serious adverse events were reported. A third review included 4 randomized studies of pharmacologic management.[29] The conclusions were similar. A fourth review included non-pharmacological and pharmacological treatments.[30] Regarding non-pharmacological approaches, the authors noted that few studies have focused on the efficacy of cognitive, emotional, or environmental interventions although they are widely used. They also noted the paucity of high-quality randomized trials of pharmacological interventions

Harms

No systematic reviews have identified harms associated with screening. Potential harms include misclassification resulting in patients either receiving unnecessary treatment or failing to receive potentially beneficial treatment. There is also the potential for psychological harm for the patient and their family when patients are misclassified. Screening tools, such as the Confusion Assessment Method (CAM), are not invasive and require little of the patient's or provider's time or effort. Although cost-effectiveness is beyond the scope of this review, costs to the health care system associated with administering and following up on screening test results should be considered.

Recommendations of Others

Despite the lack of direct evidence of a benefit of screening, some organizations have developed guidelines that recommend screening of patients or targeted screening of patients considered at risk for delirium. The 2010 National Institute for Health and Clinical Excellence (NICE) guideline on diagnosis, prevention, and management of delirium recommends assessment of risk factors for delirium in all patients when they first present to a hospital and observation of people admitted to a hospital at every opportunity for changes in the risk factors for delirium.[7,31] Risk factors cited include age 65 and older, cognitive impairment (past or present) and/or dementia, current hip fracture, and severe illness (defined as a clinical condition that is deteriorating or at risk of deteriorating). The recommendation is based on low and moderate quality evidence from prospective cohort studies. Guidelines developed by the Delirium Guidelines Development Group (Switzerland) call for "routine screening of cognitive functions and delirium, whenever possible, using standardized instruments," notably the Mini-Mental State Examination (MMSE) or Blessed Orientation-Memory-Concentration (BOMC) tests on admission and the CAM during the hospital stay. Particular emphasis was given to systematic screening in at-risk patients. The authors noted the relative lack of evidence supporting the consensus statements.[32] The British Geriatrics Society guidelines include a recommendation to identify all patients over 65 years with cognitive impairment on admission.[33] Delirium should be considered in patients with cognitive impairment and at high risk due to severe illness, dementia, fracture of the femoral neck, and visual and hearing impairment. Serial assessments are recommended in those patients to help detect the new development of delirium. This recommendation was based on evidence from high quality systematic reviews or cohort studies or extrapolated evidence from meta-analyses, systematic reviews, or randomized trials. The Australian clinical practice guideline on management of delirium recommends establishment of a structured process for screening and diagnosis of delirium in all health care settings.[25] The recommended process includes assessment of risk of delirium and cognitive function at admission with repeat testing of high risk patients (age 70 or older, pre-existing cognitive impairment, severe medical illness, depression, abnormal sodium, and visual impairment) and further assessment for delirium and/or referral if there is a decline in the cognitive assessment score. The recommendations were based on expert opinion. Clinical practice guidelines from the American College of Critical Care Medicine of the Society of Critical Care Medicine recommend routine assessment for the presence of delirium, including ICU patients.[34] The recommendation was graded B (defined as methods strong, results inconsistent, prospective randomized controlled trials with heterogeneity present).

Key Question 1a. Do these results vary by medical unit, age, gender or comorbid conditions?

We did not find any direct evidence that screening is effective regardless of the medical unit, age or gender of the patients, or their comorbid conditions.

Key Question 1b. Does screening for delirium improve clinical outcomes?

We did not find any evidence that screening for delirium improves clinical outcomes in hospitalized (including ICU) patients.

Conclusions

We identified no randomized-controlled trials of screening for delirium in hospitalized patients. We identified several studies that have compared the diagnostic accuracy of a screening tool to an established reference standard (validation studies). Most of these reports focused on selected subsets of hospitalized patients who were at high risk for delirium. Results from those studies are reported in Key Question 3. In addition, there have been many application studies (i.e., evaluating patients at admission and during their hospital stay and reporting on prevalent [present at the time of admission] and incident [developed during hospitalization] cases of delirium). A recent systematic review summarizes validation, adaptation, translation, and application studies for the CAM.[35]

Unfortunately, these types of studies do not address the question of whether screening for delirium in asymptomatic individuals improves patient outcomes nor do they directly assess the potential harms associated with universal screening. Therefore, the available evidence is insufficient to make recommendations about the net benefit of delirium screening among all hospitalized patients or patients admitted to intensive care units.

KEY QUESTION #2. What are the effectiveness and harms of delirium prevention strategies in acute elderly inpatients?

Predisposing and precipitating factors for delirium have been well documented.[4,6,36] Predisposing factors include poor nutrition, dehydration, alcohol or drug abuse, medication use (especially use of sleep medications, narcotic pain relievers, anticholinergics, sedative hypnotics, anti-depressants, Parkinson's disease treatments, anti-convulsants, muscle relaxants, and allergy medications), impaired vision or hearing, sleep deprivation, and low level of activity. Precipitating factors include infection, alcohol or drug withdrawal, emotional stress, multiple medical procedures, pain, and electrolyte disturbances. Prevention strategies typically target one or more of these factors.

Summary of Studies for Key Question 2

The study design, population and study characteristics and quality and outcomes evaluated for each of the included studies are presented in Table 1 and Appendix D, Tables 1 and 3.

Study design and location

Thirty-nine unique studies on prevention of delirium enrolling between 15 and 1059 subjects met inclusion for Key Question 2. A total of 7935 subjects were enrolled in these 39 studies.

Twenty studies evaluated pharmacologic methods for preventing delirium; sixteen of these were randomized,[13,37-51] while four were non-randomized studies.[12,52-54] Five studies evaluated cholinesterase inhibitors,[12,40,45,47,54] while four examined anesthesia,[39,41,48,51] three examined analgesic agents,[13,43,53] four examined antipsychotic medications,[38,44,46,50] and one each examined melatonin,[37] benzodiazepines,[49] post-operative sedation,[42] and a lipid-lowering agent.[52]

Nineteen studies (in 24 publications) evaluated non-pharmacologic or mixed methods of preventing delirium; five of these were randomized[55-59] and fourteen were non-randomized.[60-78] The majority of these studies evaluated multi-component interventions, often combined with staff education.[55,58-67,69-78] The multi-component interventions varied greatly and included such components as geriatric consultation, individual care planning, focused prevention of infection, improving mobility, frequent orientation, bowel and bladder care regimens, insomnia protocols, adequate pain management, minimizing psychoactive or sedating medications, and maintaining adequate hydration and nutrition, among others. Other non-pharmacologic studies examined bright light therapy,[56] the use of music,[57] or the use of staff education alone[68] as strategies for preventing delirium.

Of the 39 prevention studies of delirium, 16 were conducted in Europe, 14 in the United States, 4 in Japan, 2 in Australia, , 2 in Canada and 1 in Thailand.

Table 1. Summary of Study Baseline Characteristics for Delirium Prevention Studies

Characteristic	Mean (range) *Unless otherwise noted*	Number of trials reporting
Total number of patients evaluated	7935 (15 to 1059)	39
% of patients (n/N) in randomized pharmacologic intervention studies	28 (2245/7935)	16
% of patients (n/N) in non-randomized pharmacologic intervention studies	17 (1311/7935)	4
% of patients (n/N) in randomized non-pharmacologic intervention studies	11 (866/7935)	5
% of patients (n/N) in non-randomized non-pharmacologic intervention studies	44 (3513/7935)	14
Age of subjects, years	78 (58 to 85)	33
Gender, male, %	44 (19 to 100)	34
Race/ethnicity, white, %	91 (87 to 98)	5
Orthopedics/orthopedic surgery, % of patients (n/N)	33 (2626/7935)	15
Cardiac surgery, % of patients (n/N)	19 (1481/7935)	5
Other surgery, % of patients (n/N)	8 (673/7935)	8
Internal medicine/geriatrics/other, % of patients (n/N)	40 (3155/7935)	11
Studies conducted in the US/Canada, % of patients (n/N)	53 (4253/7935)	16
Studies conducted in Europe, % of patients (n/N)	40 (3161/7935)	16
Studies conducted in Asia/Australia, % of patients (n/N)	7% (521/7935)	7

Patient characteristics

One of the included studies enrolled U.S. veterans.[41] The mean age of the patients included in the 33 prevention studies that reported age was 78 years (range 58 to 85). Twenty-one studies enrolled only patients age 65 or greater. Men comprised 44% of subjects (range 18%-100) in the 34 studies that reported gender. Only five studies reported racial or ethnic characteristics;[38,41,47,59,71] the vast majority of subjects in those five studies were Caucasian (91%, range 87% to 98%). Twenty-eight of the studies involved patients on post-surgical units,[13,37-57,59,60,66,69,70,76] ten involved patients on medicine wards,[12,58,61,63,65,67,68,71,77,78] and one involved patients on medical-surgical units.[62]

Outcome measures

Outcomes reported varied widely between delirium prevention studies included in this report (Appendix D, Tables 2 and 4). All reported delirium incidence, with rates of delirium ranging from 11% to 88.9% in controls. Nine studies reported data regarding delirium severity. Fourteen studies reported data on delirium duration. Twenty-two studies reported data on hospital length of stay. Seven studies reported data regarding use of rescue medications.

Study quality

Most included studies assessing prevention measures utilized methods to reduce sources of bias (Appendix D, Tables 1 and 3). However, 11 studies did not report clear allocation concealment when concealment was possible. Thirteen studies did not utilize an intention-to-treat analysis (or were unclear in reporting) in studies where this would have been possible. Most studies adequately reported withdrawals from the study when this was appropriate, but three studies that would have been appropriate to report withdrawals did not do so.

Effectiveness

Pharmacologic Studies

Twenty studies evaluated pharmacologic interventions (Table 2, Appendix D, Tables 1 and 2). Most interventions were only assessed in single studies that were small in size. All but two studies[12,37] involved post-surgical patients. While all studies reported incidence, 6 reported a measure of delirium severity, 7 reported delirium duration, 11 reported length of stay, and 5 reported use of rescue medications (Appendix D, Table 2). Table 2 lists studies by intervention and provides incidence/prevalence data and relative risks.

Table 2: Incidence of Delirium – Pharmacologic Prevention Studies

Study	Study Type/Patients	Intervention / Control	Delirium Incidence/ Prevalence % (n/N)	Relative Risk [95% Confidence Interval]
Cholinesterase Inhibitors				
Liptzin, 2005[47]	RCT/orthopedic	Donepezil / Placebo	21 (8/39) / 17 (7/41)	1.20 [0.48 to 3.00]
Sampson, 2007[45]	RCT/orthopedic	Donepezil / Placebo	11 (2/19) / 36 (5/14)	0.29 [0.07 to 1.30]
Gamberini, 2009[40]	RCT/cardiac surgery	Rivastigmine / Placebo	32 (18/56) / 30 (17/57)	1.08 [0.62 to 1.87]
Dautzenberg, 2004[12]	Non-randomized/ geriatric medicine	Rivastigmine / No Rivastigmine	46 (5/11) / 89 (26/29)	0.51 [0.26 to 0.98]
Savage, 1978[54]	Non-randomized/ elective surgery	Physostigmine / No Physostigmine	9 (4/45) / 43 (29/68)	0.21 [0.08 to 0.55]
Typical Antipsychotics				
Kalisvaart, 2005[46]	RCT/orthopedic	Haloperidol / Placebo	15 (32/212) / 17 (36/218)	0.91 [0.59 to 1.42]
Kaneko, 1991[50]	RCT/gastrointestinal	Haloperidol / Placebo	11 (4/38) / 33 (13/40)	0.32 [0.12 to 0.91]
Atypical Antipsychotics				
Larsen, 2010[38]	RCT/orthopedic	Olanzapine / Placebo	14 (28/196) / 40 (82/204)	0.36 [0.24 to 0.52]
Prakanrattana, 2007[44]	RCT/cardiac surgery	Risperidone / Placebo	11 (7/63) / 32 (20/63)	0.35 [0.16 to 0.77]
Analgesia				
Mouzopolous, 2009[43]	RCT/orthopedic	Fascia iliaca compartment block / Placebo	11 (11/102) / 24 (25/105)	0.45 [0.24 to 0.87]
Williams-Russo, 1992[13]	RCT/orthopedic	Continuous epidural / Continuous intravenous analgesia	38 (10/26) / 44 (11/25)	0.87 [0.45 to 1.69]
Del Rosario, 2008[53]	Non-randomized/ orthopedic	Patient controlled, femoral nerve / Intravenous	8 (4/49) / 42 (21/50)	0.19 [0.07 to 0.53]
Anesthesia				
Papaioannou, 2005[48]	RCT/elective surgery	Regional (spinal or epidural) / General	16 (3/19) / 21 (6/28)	0.74 [0.21 to 2.59]
Berggren, 1987[51]	RCT/orthopedic	Epidural / General	50 (14/28) / 38 (11/29)	1.32 [0.73 to 2.39]
Sieber, 2010[39]	RCT/orthopedic	Light sedation / Deep sedation	19 (11/57) / 40 (23/57)	0.48 [0.26 to 0.89]
Hudetz, 2009[41]	RCT/cardiac surgery	Adjuvant Ketamine (during induction) / Placebo	3 (1/29) / 31 (9/29)	0.11 [0.02 to 0.82]
Postoperative Sedation				
Maldonado, 2009[42]	RCT/cardiac surgery	Dexmedetomidine / Propofol	10 (4/40) / 44 (16/36)	0.23 [0.08 to 0.61]
Maldonado, 2009[42]	RCT/cardiac surgery	Dexmedetomidine / Midazolam	10 (4/40) / 43 (17/40)	0.24 [0.09 to 0.64]
Delirium Free Protocol				
Aizawa, 2002[49]	RCT/gastrointestinal	Benzodiazepines+Pethidine / Usual care	5 (1/20) / 35 (7/20)	0.14 [0.02 to 1.06]
Melatonin				
Al-Aama, 2011[37]	RCT/internal medicine	Melatonin / Placebo	11 (7/61) / 31 (19/61)	0.37 [0.17 to 0.81]
Anti-Lipid Therapy				
Katznelson, 2009[52]	Non-randomized/ cardiac surgery	Statin / No statin	11 (73/676) / 13 (49/383)	0.84 [0.60 to 1.19]

Of the five studies evaluating cholinesterase inhibitors, two non-randomized trials found that using cholinesterase inhibitors was an effective strategy for decreasing the incidence of delirium. One study compared hospitalized patients who were chronic users of rivastigmine to non-users and found a decreased incidence of delirium in the chronic users (N=40, 45.5% vs. 88.9%, p=0.007).[12] The second study compared delirium incidence in elective surgery patients given physostigmine or placebo (N=113, 28.9% vs. 69.1%, p=0.0004).[54] Three randomized, controlled trials found no difference in delirium incidence between intervention and control subjects using rivastigmine in cardiac surgery patients (N=120, 32.1% vs. 29.8%, p=0.79)[40] or donepezil in hip replacement patients (N=50, 10.5% vs. 35.7%, p=0.08)[45] and hip and knee replacement patients (N=80, 20.5% vs. 17.1%, p=0.69).[47] There were no reported differences between intervention and control groups in delirium severity, delirium duration, hospital length of stay, or use of rescue medications.

Four studies looked at different anesthesia protocols. One study found that limiting the depth of intra-operative sedation during spinal anesthesia for hip fracture repair decreased the incidence of delirium in subjects receiving light sedation vs. subjects receiving deep sedation (N=114, 19% vs. 40%, p=0.02).[39] This intervention was also found to decrease delirium duration (0.5 days (SD 1.5) vs. 1.4 days (SD 4.0), p=0.01), but did not have a significant effect on delirium severity or hospital length of stay. In veterans undergoing elective cardiac surgery with cardiopulmonary bypass, ketamine (vs. saline) during anesthetic induction significantly reduced the incidence of delirium (N=58, 3.4% vs. 31.0%, p=0.01)[41] Length of stay did not differ. A small, single site study comparing regional (epidural or spinal) anesthesia to general anesthesia in patients undergoing elective orthopedic or vascular surgery found no difference in the incidence of delirium (N=47, 15.8% vs. 21.4%, p=0.63).[48] Similarly, in another small study there was no significant difference in the incidence of delirium in patients receiving epidural vs. general anesthesia during femoral neck fracture repair (N=57, 50% vs. 27.9%, p=0.36).[51]

Of the four studies evaluating antipsychotic medications, all involved surgical patients. Three found a significantly lower incidence of delirium in the intervention groups compared to the control groups[38,44,50] The studies all compared use of prophylactic antipsychotics to that of placebo; one used olanzapine perioperatively in patients undergoing total knee or hip replacement (N=495, 14.3% vs. 40.2%, p<0.0001),[38] one used risperidone following elective cardiac surgery with cardiopulmonary bypass (N=126, 11.1% vs. 31.7%, p=0.009),[44] and one use haloperidol following gastrointestinal surgery(N=80, 10.5% vs 32.5%, p<0.05).[50] A more recent study of haloperidol for patients undergoing elective hip surgery found no difference (N=430, 15.1% vs. 16.5%, p=0.69).[46] The study using olanzapine also found a decrease in delirium severity (DRS-R-98 score of 16.4 (SD 3.7) vs. 14.5 (SD 2.7), p=0.002) and duration (2.2 days (SD 1.3) vs. 1.6 (SD 0.7), p=0.02) in the treatment group;[38] these outcomes were not reported in the study using risperidone[44] or in one of the haloperidol studies[50] The second haloperidol study reported significant decreases in severity and duration of delirium (both p<0.01) and a difference in length of stay for patient who developed delirium (11.1 days vs. 16.7 days, p<0.001)[46]

Of the three studies evaluating analgesia, two studies found enhanced pain prophylaxis decreased delirium incidence. One studied used a fascia iliaca compartment block (injection of local anesthesia beneath the fascial layer of the iliopsoas muscle as an approach to reaching the nerves of the lumbar plexus) vs. placebo before and after hip fracture surgery (N=219, 10.8%

vs. 23.8%, p=0.02).[43] The other study, a retrospective comparison of patients who received patient-controlled femoral nerve analgesia vs. intravenous analgesia following hip fracture surgery (N=99, 8.2% vs. 42.0%, p<0.001).[53] A third study did not find a difference in delirium incidence between intervention subjects using continuous epidural bupivicaine and fentanyl vs. control subjects using continuous IV fentanyl for pain following bilateral knee replacement (N=51, 38.4% vs. 44.0%, p=0.69).[13] The study using the fascia iliaca compartment block[43] found significant differences in delirium severity (DRS-R-98 score of 14.3 (SD 3.6) vs. 18.6 (3.4), p<0.001) and duration (5.2 days (SD 4.3) vs. 11.0 days (SD 7.2), p<0.001) favoring the treatment intervention. The study using the patient-controlled femoral nerve analgesia[53] found a significant difference in use of opioid rescue medications favoring the intervention group (0% vs. 28%, p<0.001).

Other pharmacologic agents studied include melatonin, bendodiazipines, other post-operative sedatives, and anti-lipids. A recent study of melatonin prior to sleep in patients on the internal medicine wards found a decreased incidence of delirium compared to patients receiving placebo (N=122, 11.5% vs. 31.1%, p=0.01).[37] Post-operative sedation with dexmedetomidine compared to either propofol or midazolam following cardiac valve surgery (with cardiopulmonary bypass) resulted in a decreased incidence of delirium (N=76, dexmedetomidine 10.0%, propofol 44.4%, midazolam 42.5%, p<0.001 dexmedetomidine vs. both controls).[42] There were also no differences in delirium duration, length of stay, or use of rescue medications.[42] A study of a delirium-free protocol (diazepam, flunitrazepam, and pethidine) vs. usual care in patients who underwent resection of gastric or colorectal cancer found no difference in the incidence of delirium (N=40, 5.0% vs. 35.0%, p=0.06).[49] Length of stay also did not differ. A non-randomized study found that administration of anti-lipid therapy did not alter the development of delirium between intervention and control subjects following cardiac surgery (N=1059, 10.8% vs.12.8%, p=0.33).[52]

Pooled Comparisons (Figure 5)

We were able to pool randomized trials of antipsychotics versus placebo studies and cholinesterase inhibitors versus placebo for analysis; the other pharmacologic trials were too heterogeneous to allow for meta-analysis. In three small trials of cholinesterase inhibitor medications versus placebo (combined n = 226),[40,45,47] prophylactic cholinesterase inhibitors (donepezil and rivastigimine) did not significantly decrease the development of delirium in older hospitalized patients (RR 0.93, 95%CI 0.51-1.69, I^2=29%).

In two trials of atypical antipsychotic medication versus placebo involving 526 individuals,[38,44] prophylactic medications significantly decreased the development of delirium in older hospitalized patients (RR 0.35, 95%CI 0.25-0.50, I^2=0%).

Strength of Evidence (Table 3)

We evaluated the strength of evidence for the randomized studies of pharmacologic interventions using the approach described in the Methods section. Strength of evidence was low for all of the interventions that included only one randomized trial. Study quality, reflecting risk of bias, was rated as fair for all but one of the studies. Imprecision was noted for five of the studies. With one trial, it was not possible to assess consistency of the intervention effect.

For the two comparisons with multiple trials, one was rated low (acetylcholinesterase inhibitors versus placebo) while one was rated moderate (atypical antipsychotic agents versus placebo). Overall study quality was fair for both interventions but precision and consistency were noted for the atypical antipsychotic trials.

Figure 5. Incidence of Delirium, Randomized Pharmacologic Trials

A. Acetylcholinesterase inhibitors versus placebo

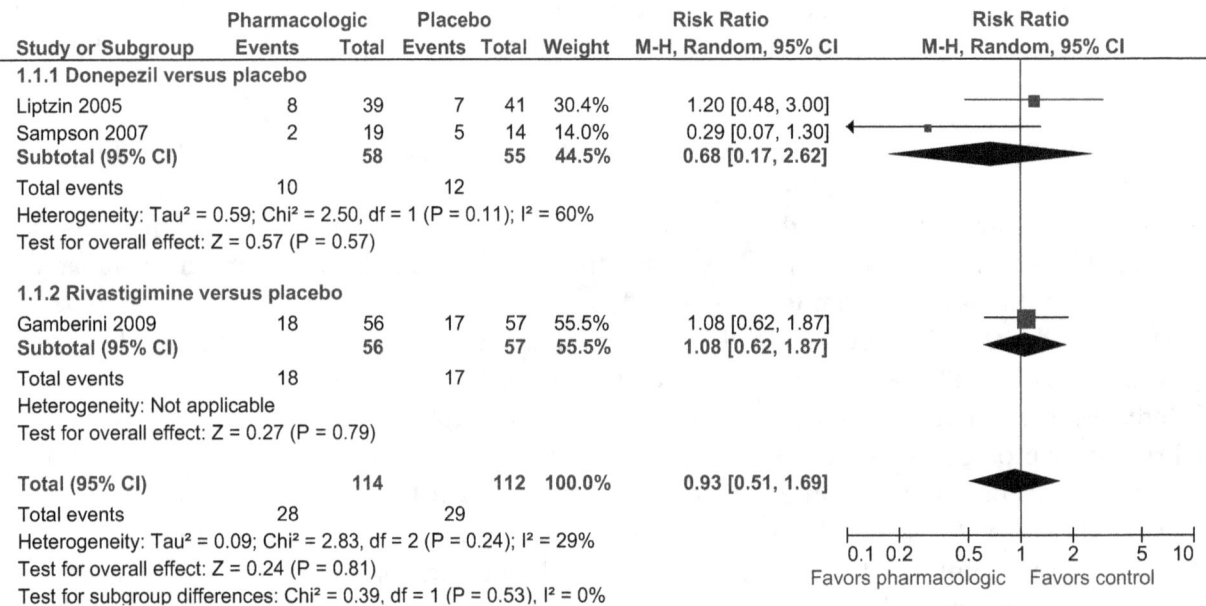

B. Atypical antipsychotic agents versus placebo

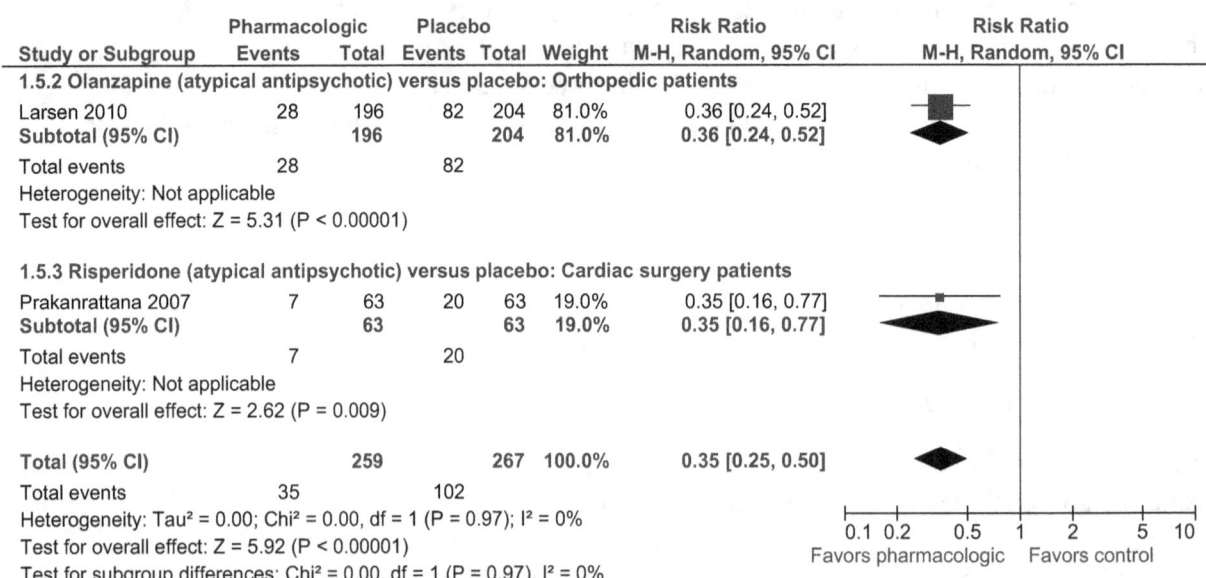

Table 3. Evidence Summaries for the Randomized Pharmacologic Delirium Studies: Incidence of Delirium

Intervention	Meta-analysis details; notes	Summary statistics	Quality domains	Evidence rating
Acetylcholinesterase inhibitors versus placebo Liptzin 2005; Sampson 2007; Gamberini 2009)[40,45,47]	3 trials (n=226) agents: donepezil (2) and rivastigimine	RR = 0.93 [95%CI 0.51 to 1.69]	Study quality: fair Directness: direct Imprecision: yes Inconsistency: yes	Low
Atypical antipsychotic agents versus placebo (Larsen 2010; Prakanrattana 2007)[38,44]	2 trials (n=526) agents: olanzapine and risperidone	RR = 0.32 [95%CI 0.12 to 0.91]	Study quality: fair Directness: direct Imprecision: no Inconsistency: no	Moderate
Typical antipsychotic agents versus placebo (with consultation) (Kalisvaart 2005)[46]	1 trial (n=430) proactive geriatric consultation for all patients agent: haloperidol	RR = 0.91 [95%CI 0.59 to 1.42]	Study quality: good Directness: direct Imprecision: yes Inconsistency: NA	Low
Typical antipsychotic agents versus placebo (Kaneko 1999)[50]	1 trial (n=78) agent: haloperidol	RR = 0.32 [95%CI 0.12 to 0.91]	Study quality: fair Directness: direct Imprecision: no Inconsistency: NA	Low
Fascia iliaca block versus placebo (Mouzopolous 2009)[43] *Analgesia*	1 trial (n=207)	RR = 0.45 [95%CI 0.24 to 0.87]	Study quality: fair Directness: direct Imprecision: no Inconsistency: NA	Low
Continuous epidural versus continuous intravenous (Williams-Russo 1992)[13] *Analgesia*	1 trial (n=51)	RR = 0.87 [95%CI 0.45 to 1.69]	Study quality: fair Directness: direct Imprecision: yes Inconsistency: NA	Low
Deep sedation versus light sedation (Sieber 2010)[39] *Anesthesia*	1 trial (n=114) agent: propofol	RR = 0.48 [95%CI 0.26 to 0.89]	Study quality: fair Directness: direct Imprecision: no Inconsistency: NA	Low
Ketamine bolus versus placebo (Hudetz 2009)[41] *Anesthesia*	1 trial (n=58) administered during anesthetic induction	RR = 0.11 [95%CI 0.02 to 0.82]	Study quality: fair Directness: direct Imprecision: no Inconsistency: NA	Low

21

Intervention	Meta-analysis details; notes		Summary statistics	Quality domains	Evidence rating
Regional anesthesia versus general anesthesia (Papaioannou 2005)[48] *Anesthesia*	1 trial	regional was either epidural or spinal	RR = 0.74 [95%CI 0.21 to 2.59]	Study quality: fair	Low
	(n=47)			Directness: direct	
				Imprecision: yes	
				Inconsistency: NA	
Epidural anesthesia versus general anesthesia (Berggren 1987)[51] *Anesthesia*			RR = 1.32 [95%CI 0.73 to 2.39]	Study quality: fair	Low
	(n=57)			Directness: direct	
				Imprecision: yes	
				Inconsistency: NA	
Postoperative dexmedetomidine Sedation versus postoperative propofol sedation (Maldonado 2009)[42]	1 trial		RR = 0.23 [95%CI 0.08 to 0.61]	Study quality: fair	Low
	(n=76)			Directness: direct	
				Imprecision: no	
				Inconsistency: NA	
Postoperative dexmedetomidine Sedation versus postoperative midazolam sedation (Maldonado 2009)[42]	1 trial		RR = 0.24 [95%CI 0.09 to 0.64]	Study quality: fair	Low
	(n=80)			Directness: direct	
				Imprecision: no	
				Inconsistency: NA	
Delirium free protocol (DFP) versus usual care (Aizawa 2002)[49]	1 trial	DFP: benzodiazepines and pethidine	RR = 0.14 [95%CI 0.02 to 1.06]	Study quality: fair	Low
	(n=40)			Directness: direct	
				Imprecision: yes	
				Inconsistency: NA	
Melatonin versus placebo (Al-Aama 2011)[37]	1 trial		RR = 0.37 [95%CI 0.17 to 0.81]	Study quality: fair	Low
	(n=122)			Directness: direct	
				Imprecision: no	
				Inconsistency: NA	

The remaining nonrandomized studies (Katznelson 2009, anti-lipid therapy;[52] Del Rosario 2008, analgesia;[53] Dautzenberg 2004 and Savage 1978, both acetylcholinesterase inhibitors[12,54]) should be considered at high-risk of bias due to lower study quality and therefore the summary of evidence is low.

CI = confidence interval; NA = not applicable; RR = relative risk

Non-Pharmacologic or Mixed Studies

Nineteen studies, including 5 randomized, controlled trials and 14 non-randomized trials, evaluated non-pharmacologic or mixed methods of delirium prevention (Tables 4 and 5, Appendix D, Tables 3 and 4). Included patients tended to be at moderate-to-high risk for delirium, with patients recruited post-operatively, from ICUs or traumatological unit, or as geriatric internal medicine patients. The studies were widely variable in their interventions and reporting of outcomes. All reported on some measure of delirium incidence, 4 studies reported delirium severity, 7 studies reported delirium duration, 11 studies reported length of stay, and 2 studies reported on the use of rescue medications). Of the 5 randomized trials, one assessed music therapy, one bright light therapy, one proactive geriatrics consultation and two involved staff education and varying multi-component interventions.

Sixteen of the nineteen non-pharmacologic prevention studies examined multi-component interventions (see Table 4). Authors reported a significantly lower incidence of delirium in the intervention group in 2 of the 3 randomized trials and 10 of the 12 non-randomized trials (p<0.05) with one trial not reporting the significance level (Appendix D, Table 2). When relative risks were determined, all but one study found a reduced risk of delirium in the intervention; the difference was significant in 1 of the 3 randomized trials and 6 of the 12 non-randomized trials (Table 5). Relative risks in the 3 randomized trials ranged from 0.65 to 1.01; in the 12 non-randomized trials, the range was 0.16 to 0.88. Of four multi-component studies reporting delirium severity, two reported that the intervention decreased severity.[65,70] Three of seven studies reporting decreased delirium duration reported significantly better outcomes in the intervention group.[55,70,71] Of eleven studies reporting length of stay, four found significantly shorter hospitalization for intervention patients with differences of 4 to 10 days.[55,58,66,78] Both of the studies reporting on rescue medication use with found reductions among intervention patients.[55,67]

Three non-pharmacologic studies used a single intervention prevention strategy including randomized trials of bright light therapy[56] and music[57] and a non-randomized study of staff education alone.[68] Using bright lights to enhance daytime awakening was not found to be an effective prevention strategy for delirium (N=15, 16.7% vs. 40.0%, p=0.42),[56] however, playing largely instrumental, soothing music four times per day significantly decreased delirium incidence (N=126, 3.2% vs. 58.1%, p=0.001).[57] A third study found that educating staff to increase delirium awareness and knowledge was effective in decreasing delirium incidence (N=250, 9.8% vs. 19.5%, p=0.03).[68] None of these studies reported on other delirium outcomes.

Pooled Comparisons

The non-pharmacologic or mixed delirium prevention strategies could not be pooled due to the heterogeneity of the interventions tested.

Strength of Evidence (Table 6)

We determined strength of evidence for the five randomized trials of non-pharmacologic interventions. One study was rated moderate due to the higher quality (lower risk of bias) of the study; the remaining four were rated low. Due to heterogeneity of the interventions, we did not rate the strength of evidence for the non-randomized trials.

Table 4. Components of Multi-Component Interventions for Delirium Prevention

Study/Patients	Multi-Disciplinary Team	Staff Education	Patient Assessment	Orientation and/or Sensory Impairment Training	Sleep Protocol	Early Mobilization	Environmental Modification	Medication Modification/Pain Management	Nutrition/Hydration
Randomized Controlled Trials									
Lundstrom 2007[55]/orthopedic (other-individual care planning, bowel/bladder function, oxygen)	✓	✓	✓		✓	✓		✓	✓
Lundstrom 2005[58]/internal medicine (items covered in nurse and staff training)		✓	✓	✓				✓	
Marcantonio 2001[59]/orthopedic (other – oxygen, bowel/bladder function)			✓	✓		✓	✓	✓	✓
Non-randomized Trials									
Ushida 2009[60]/neurology			✓	✓	✓	✓		✓	
Vidan 2009[61]/internal medicine	✓	✓	✓	✓	✓	✓		✓	✓
Kratz 2008[62]/medical-surgical	✓	✓	✓	✓	✓	✓	✓	✓	✓
Robinson 2008,[63] Vollmer 2007[64]/renal	✓	✓	✓	✓		✓	✓		
Caplan 2007[65]/geriatrics			✓	✓					✓
Harari 2007[66]/orthopedic (other-bowel/bladder function, discharge planning)	✓		✓			✓		✓	✓
Naughton 2005[67]/medicine	✓	✓	✓		✓	✓	✓	✓	
Wong Tim Niam 2005[69]/orthopedic (other-bladder/bowel function, oxygen)		✓	✓	✓		✓	✓	✓	✓
Milisen 2001[70]/traumatologic		✓	✓					✓	
Inouye 1999[71] and 4 related publications[72-75]/general medicine	✓	✓	✓	✓	✓	✓			✓
Lundstrom 1999[76]/orthopedic (other-oxygen)	✓	✓	✓		✓	✓	✓		✓
Wanich 1992[77]/general medicine (other-discharge planning, caregiver education)	✓	✓	✓	✓		✓	✓	✓	
Gustafson 1991[78]/orthopedic (other-surgery policy, oxygen, anesthetic technique)	✓		✓						

Table 5: Incidence of Delirium - Non-Pharmacologic or Mixed Treatments Prevention Studies

Study	Study Type/Patients	Intervention / Control	Delirium Incidence/ Prevalence % (n/N)	Relative Risk [95% Confidence Interval]
Lundstrom, 2007[55]	RCT/orthopedic	Multi-factorial intervention / Usual care	55 (56/102) / 75 (73/97)	0.73 [0.59 to 0.90]
Taguchi, 2007[56]	RCT/ICU	Bright light therapy / Natural lighting environment	17 (1/6) / 40 (2/5)	0.42 [0.05 to 3.36]
McCaffrey, 2006[57]	RCT/orthopedic	Music plus usual care / Usual care	3 (2/62) / 58 (36/62)	0.06 [0.01 to 0.22]
Lundstrom, 2005[58]	RCT/general medicine	Multi-component including education / Usual care	32 (63/200) / 31 (62/200)	1.01 [0.76 to 1.36]
Marcantonio, 2001[59]	RCT/orthopedic	Proactive geriatrics consultation / Usual care	32 (20/62) / 50 (32/64)	0.65 [0.42 to 1.00]
Ushida, 2009[60]	Non-randomized/ neurology	Modified protocol / Usual care	8 (3/38) / 28 (23/81)	0.28 [0.09 to 0.87]
Vidan, 2009[61]	Non-randomized/ geriatric medicine	Multi-disciplinary/component intervention / Usual care	12 (20/170) / 19 (69/372)	0.63 [0.40 to 1.01]
Robinson, 2008[63,64]	Non-randomized/ renal	Delirium protocol / Usual care	14 (11/80) / 38 (30/80)	0.37 [0.20 to 0.68]
Caplan, 2007[65]	Non-randomized/ geriatric	Multi-component intervention / Usual care	6 (1/16) / 38 (8/21)	0.16 [0.02 to 1.18]
Harari, 2007[66]	Non-randomized/ orthopedic	Proactive care of older people (POPS) / Pre-POPS	6 (3/54) / 19 (10/54)	0.30 [0.09 to 1.03]
Naughton, 2005[67] 4-month cohort	Non-randomized/ geriatric or general med	Multi-factorial intervention / Pre-intervention strategy	23 (35/154) / 41 (45/110)	0.56 [0.38 to 0.80]
Naughton, 2005[67] 9-month cohort	Non-randomized/ geriatric or general med	Multi-factorial intervention / Pre-intervention strategy	19 (21/110) / 41 (45/110)	0.47 [0.30 to 0.73]
Tabet, 2005[68]	Non-randomized/ medicine	Educational package / No educational package	10 (12/122) / 20 (25/128)	0.50 [0.26 to 0.96]
Wong Tim Niam, 2005[69]	Non-randomized/ orthopedic	Quality improvement program / No program group	13 (9/71) / 36 (10/28)	0.35 [0.16 to 0.78]
Milisen, 2001[70]	Non-randomized/ traumatological ward	Education of nursing staff / Usual care	20 (12/60) / 23 (14/60)	0.86 [0.46 to 1.45]
Inouye, 1999[71-75]	Non-randomized/ general medicine	Multi-component strategy / Matched controls	10 (42/426) / 15 (64/426)	0.66 [0.46 to 0.95]
Lundstrom, 1999[76]	Non-randomized/ orthopedic	Multi-component/education / Usual care or medical intervention	31 (15/49) / 55 (117/214)	0.56 [0.36 to 0.87]
Wanich, 1992[77]	Non-randomized/ general medicine	Multi-component/education / Usual care	19 (26/135) / 22 (22/100)	0.88 [0.53 to 1.45]
Gustafson, 1991[78]	Non-randomized/ orthopedic	Surgical/anesthesia policy / Pre-surgical/anesthesia policy	48 (49/103) / 61 (68/111)	0.78 [0.60 to 1.00]

RCT = randomized controlled trial

Table 6. Evidence Summaries for the Randomized Non-pharmacologic Delirium Studies: Incidence of Delirium

Intervention	Meta-analysis details; notes	Summary statistics	Quality domains	Evidence rating
Multi-factorial intervention (postoperative) program versus usual care (Lundstrom 2007)[55] *Orthopedics*	1 trial (n=199) program elements included: a) multi-disciplinary team; b) staff education; c) patient assessment; d) sleep protocol; e) early mobilization; f) medication modification/pain management; g) nutrition/hydration	RR = 0.73 [0.59 to 0.90]	Study quality: good Directness: direct Imprecision: no Inconsistency: NA	Moderate
Multi-component intervention versus usual care (Lundstrom 2005)[58] *Internal medicine*	1 trial (n=400) program elements included: a) staff education; b) patient assessment; c) orientation and/or sensory impairment training; d) medication modification/pain management	RR = 1.01 [0.76 to 1.36]	Study quality: fair Directness: direct Imprecision: no Inconsistency: NA	Low
Multi-component intervention (proactive geriatrics consultation (preoperatively or within 24 hours of surgery) versus usual care (Marcantonio 2001)[59] *Orthopedics*	1 trial (n=126) program elements included: a) patient assessment; b) orientation and/or sensory impairment training; c) early mobilization; d) environmental modification; f) nutrition/hydration	RR = 0.65 [0.42 to 1.00]	Study quality: fair Directness: direct Imprecision: yes Inconsistency: NA	Low
Bright light therapy versus Natural lighting environment (Taguchi 2007)[56] *ICU,*	1 trial (n=15) patients undergoing surgery for esophageal cancer	RR = 0.42 [0.05 to 3.36]	Study quality: fair-poor Directness: direct Imprecision: yes Inconsistency: NA	Low
Usual post-operative care plus music versus usual post-operative care (McCaffrey 2006)[57] *Orthopedics*	1 trial (n=126) patient's choice from CDs provided	RR = 0.06 [0.01 to 0.22]	Study quality: fair-poor Directness: direct Imprecision: no Inconsistency: NA	Low

The remaining nonrandomized studies should be considered at high-risk of bias due to lower study quality and therefore the summary of evidence is low.

CI = confidence interval; ICU = intensive care unit; NA = not applicable; RR = relative risk

Harms

Mortality and adverse event data are reported on Table 7. Only trials reporting adverse event or mortality data are listed. Due to incomplete reporting and widely varying level of detail among studies that did report, it is difficult to determine whether one type of intervention was more likely to result in adverse events or deaths.

Mortality

Seven studies of pharmacological interventions and eleven studies of non-pharmacological interventions report mortality data. Only one study, using a multi-component intervention, reported a difference in mortality between intervention and control groups. For patients who developed delirium, a lower mortality rate was found in the intervention group versus the control group (2 deaths in 63 intervention subjects ([3.2%] versus 9 deaths in 62 control subjects [14.5%], p=0.03).[58]

Adverse Events

Reporting of adverse events varied. Thirteen of twenty pharmacologic intervention studies and seven of nineteen non-pharmacologic intervention studies reported adverse event data. Overall, few differences between intervention and control groups were found. Among studies of pharmacologic interventions, the only significant adverse event related to use of restraints. One study of patients admitted to internal medicine units from the emergency department found that fewer patients treated with melatonin required restraints (6.6% vs. 9.8%, p=0.03).[37] A second study, with patients who underwent elective total knee or total hip replacement surgery and received either olanzapine or placebo, found increased use of restraints in the intervention group (2.6% vs. 0%, p=0.03).[38]

Among studies of non-pharmacologic interventions, four studies reported significant differences in adverse events. One study, comparing a multi-factorial intervention to usual care in orthopedic patients, found fewer bed sores (9% vs. 22%) urinary tract infections (31% vs. 51%), nutritional complications (25% vs. 38%), and falls (12% vs. 27%) in the intervention group (all p<05).[55] A second study, before and after implementation of a multidisciplinary program for patients undergoing elective orthopedic surgery, reported decreased uncontrolled pain (2% vs. 30%) and pressure sores (4% vs. 19%), and fewer patients with bedridden status (9% s. 28%) or unable to perform independent transfers on the third post-operative day (0% vs. 15%) (all p<0.05).[66] Another pre-post study found fewer pressure sores (4% vs. 13%) and fewer severe falls (0% vs. 5%) (both p<0.05) in patients undergoing surgery for hip fractures.[78]. Finally, implementation of a multi-component protocol in the medical-surgical unit was associated with a "statistically significant" reduction in restraint use.[62]

Table 7. Adverse Events and Mortality – Prevention Studies

Author, Year	Adverse Events n/N (%)		Mortality n/N (%)	
	Intervention	Control	Intervention	Control
Pharmacologic Treatments				
Randomized trials				
Al-Aama 2011[37]	Two patients on melatonin reported side effects that might have been secondary to the study medication or related to delirium directly (1 patient reported nightmares and 1 patient reported feeling like he was "floating around and talking to his dead wife") *Clinical interventions* Restraints 4/61 (6.6), p=0.03 Use of paid attendant services 2/57 (4 missing) (3.5)	*Clinical interventions* Restraints 6/61 (9.8) Use of paid attendant services 1/60 (1 missing) (1.7)	6/61 (9.8), p=0.78 Plus additional deaths from patients excluded from study analyses (n not reported)	8/61 (13.1) Plus additional deaths from patients excluded from study analyses (n not reported)
Larsen 2010[38]	Atrial fibrillation 6/196 (3.1), p=NS Arrhythmia 2/196 (1.0), p=NS Congestive heart failure 1/196 (0.5), p=NS Alcohol withdrawal 5/196 (1.0), p=NS Pneumonia 3/196 (1.5), p=NS Urinary tract infection 1/196 (0.5%), p=NS *Clinical interventions* Sitter 9/196 (4.6), p=NS Restraints 5/196 (2.6), p=0.03 Bed alarm 11/196 (5.6), p=NS	Atrial fibrillation 3/204 (1.5) Arrhythmia 1/204 (0.5) Congestive heart failure 1 /204 (0.5) Alcohol withdrawal 1 /204 (0.5) Pneumonia 0/204(0) Urinary tract infection 4/204 (2.0) *Clinical interventions* Sitter 4/204 (2.0) Restraints 0/204 Bed alarm 7/204 (3.4)		
Sieber 2010[39]	Deep sedation Patients ≥ 1 complication 30/57 (52.6), p=0.57 Patients with postoperative complications (averaged over the entire population of each group include the following: urinary tract infection, discharge with urinary drainage catheter, acute renal failure, pneumonia, congestive heart failure, myocardial infarction, new dysrhythmia, fall, return to surgery, pulmonary embolus or deep venous thrombosis, or wound infection) 1.0 (1.8), p=NS	Light sedation Patients ≥ 1 complication 26/57 (45.6) Patients with postoperative complications (averaged over the entire population of each group) 0.8 (1.4)	Deep sedation Intraoperative 0/57, p>0.99 During hospitalization 2/57 (3.5), p>0.99	Light sedation Intraoperative 0/57 During hospitalization 1/57 (1.8)

Author, Year	Adverse Events n/N (%)		Mortality n/N (%)	
	Intervention	Control	Intervention	Control
Gamberini 2009[40]	Perioperative stroke 1/59 (1.7), p=1.0 Seizures 0/59, p=1.0 Nausea 40/59 (67.8), p=0.1 Vomiting 27/59 (45.8), p=0.6 Anorexia 39/59 (66.1), p=1.0 Diarrhea 7/59 (11.9), p=0.8 Vertigo 28/59 (47.5), p=0.5 Insomnia 33/59 (55.9), p=0.1 Atrial fibrillation 22/59 (37.3), p=0.6 Life-threatening arrhythmia 3/59 (5.1), p=1.0 Pacemaker >1 day 15/59 (25.4), p=0.12	Perioperative stroke 2/61 (3.3) Seizures 1/61 (1.6) Nausea 32/61 (52.5) Vomiting 24/61 (39.3) Anorexia 41/61 (67.2) Diarrhea 6/61 (9.8) Vertigo 24/61 (39.3) Insomnia 24/61 (39.3) Atrial fibrillation 26/61 (42.6) Life-threatening arrhythmia 3/61 (4.9) Pacemaker >1 day 24/61 (39.3)	1/59 (1.7), p=1.0	1/61 (1.6)
Maldonado 2009[42]	Postoperative hypotension 2/40 (5.0)	Midazolam group Inoperative CVA 1/40 (2.5)	0/40 Dexmedetomidine	2/38 (5.3) Propofol 0/40 Midazolam
Mouzopolous 2009[43]	3 local hematomas developed at the injection site which "resolved spontaneously", p=NR		1/108 (0.9), p=NR	2/111 (1.8)
Sampson 2007[45]	Nausea 6/19 (31.6), p=0.5 Vomiting 3/19 (15.8), p=0.5 Diarrhea 3/19 (15.8), p=0.9 Insomnia 9/19 (47.4), p=0.2 Dizziness 4/19 (21.1), p=0.3 Paresthesia 1/19 (5.3), p=0.8 Fever 1/19 (5.3), p=0.8 Subjects with 1 AE 1/19 (5.3), p=0.4 Subjects with 2 AE 17/19 (89.5), p=0.4	Nausea 6/14 (42.9) Vomiting 1/14 (7.1) Diarrhea 2/19 (10.5) Insomnia 10/19 (52.6) Dizziness 1/14 (7.1) Paresthesia 1/14 (7.1) Fever 1/14 (7.1) Subjects with 1 AE 2/14 (14.3) Subjects with 2 AE 11/14 (78.6)		
Kalisvaart 2005[46]	3 subjects withdrew due to adverse events No drug-related side effects were observed during study period.	3 subjects withdrew due to adverse events		
Papaioannou 2005[48]	Postoperative complications 5/19 (26.3), p=NS	Postoperative complications 8/28 (28.6)		
Aizawa 2002[49]	Surgical complications 5/20 (25.0) Morning lethargy 8/20 (40.0)	Surgical complications 5/20 (25.0)		
Williams-Russo 1992[13]	Complications not reported by treatment arm. Thrombocytopenia 20/51 (39.2) Atrial arrhythmias 11/51 (21.6) Hyponatremia 11/51 (21.6) Urinary tract infections 3/51 (5.9)			

Author, Year	Adverse Events n/N (%)		Mortality n/N (%)	
	Intervention	Control	Intervention	Control
Berggren 1987[51]	Pneumonia 1/28 (3.6) Pulmonary embolism 2/28 (7.1) Cardiac failure 2/28 (7.1) Depression 3/28 (10.7) Urinary incontinence 6/28 (21.4) Urinary retention 5/28 (17.9) Urinary tract infection 9/28 (32.1) Urosepsis 1/28 (3.6) Decubitus ulcer 3/28 (10.7) Stroke 3/28 (10.7) All comparisons p=NS	Pneumonia 2/29 (6.9) Depression 3/29 (10.3) Urinary incontinence 5/29 (17.2) Urinary retention 6/29 (20.7) Urinary tract infection 7/29 (24.1) Decubitus ulcer 5/29 (17.2)	One death on the first postoperative day. 3 additional deaths (group not defined) within 5 months post surgery	See intervention
Non-randomized trials				
Del Rosario 2008[53]	No statistically significant differences (p>0.05) in the transfusion index, hemoglobin level and rate of medical postoperative complications.			
Dautzenberg 2004[12]			0/11, p>0.05	0/29
Savage 1987[54]				
Non-Pharmacologic Studies				
Randomized trials				
Lundstrom 2007[55]	During hospitalization (significant differences vs. control*) Bedsores 9/102 (8.8), p=0.01 Urinary tract infection 32/102 (31.4), p=0.01 Nutritional complications 25/102 (24.5), p=0.04 Falls 12/102 (11.8), p=0.01	During hospitalization Bedsores 21/95 (22.1) Urinary tract infection 49/96 (51.0) Nutritional complications 37/97 (38.1) Falls 26/97 (26.8)	Over 12-month follow-up: 16/102 (15.7), p=NS	Over 12-month follow-up: 18/97 (18.6)
Taguchi 2007[56]	A few patients had to be reintubated (numbers not provided)			
Lundstrom 2005[58]			Delirium patients 2/63 (3.2) p=0.03	Delirium patients 9/62 (14.5)
Non-randomized trials				
Vidan 2009[61]			10/170 (5.8) Delirium patients 2/20 (10.0), p=0.60	19/372 (5.1) Delirium patients 10/69 (14.5)
Kratz 2008[62]	After implementation of acute confusion (AC) protocol Fall rate per 1000 patient days: 3.6 (in 2005); 3.6 (in 2006); 4.2 (in 2007), p=NR Restraint episodes per 1000 patient days: 1.3 (in 2005); 1.4 (in 2006); 0.09 (in 2007), reported to be "statistically significant"	Prior to implementation of AC protocol (2004) Fall rate per 1000 patient days: 4.8 Restraint episodes per 1000 patient days: 8.7		

...nIn Screening, Prevention, and Diagnosis: A Systematic Review of the Evidence

Author, Year	Adverse Events n/N (%)		Mortality n/N (%)	
	Intervention	Control	Intervention	Control
Caplan 2007[65]			0/16, p=NR	1/21 (4.8)
Harari 2007[66]	Uncontrolled pain: 1/54 (1.9), p<0.01 No food for ≥ 4 days post-op: 0/54 Pressure sores: 2/54 (3.7), p=0.03 Bedridden: 5/54 (9.3), p=0.01 Dependent transfers on day 3 post-op: 0/54, p<0.01	Uncontrolled pain: 16/54 (29.6) No food for ≥ 4 days: 5/54 (9.3) Pressure sores: 10/54 (18.5) Bedridden: 15/54 (27.8) Dependent transfers on day 3 post-op: 8/54 (14.8)	0/54, p=NR	1/54 (1.9)
Wong Tim Niam 2005[69]			Baseline period 2/28 (7.1), p=NR	Post-intervention 3/71 (4.2)
Milisen 2001[70]			Small number of deaths in the sample OR for death in intervention cohort vs. non-intervention cohort: 3.86 (95%CI 0.09-1.71)	
Inouye 1999[71]			6/426 (1.4) p=0.78	7/426 (1.6)
Lundstrom 1999[76]	Severe falls 0/49 p=0.10 vs. C1 Eating problems 1/49 (2.0) p=0.19 vs. C1	Severe falls Control 1 6/111 (5.4) Control 2 0/103 Eating problems Control 1 8/111 (7.2) Control 2 5/103 (4.9)	In-hospital 1/49 (2.0) p=0.81vs. C1, p=0.30 vs. C2 6-month 8/49 (16.3) p=0.99 vs. C1, p=0.54 vs. C2	In-hospital Control 1 3/111 (2.7) Control 2 6/103 (5.8) 6-month Control 1 18/111 (16.2) Control 2 13/103 (12.6)
Wanich 1992[77]	Complications: 25/135 (19.0), p=NS (at least 1 of 11 pre-defined events that developed in-hospital)	Complications: 16/100 (16.0)	Hospital mortality: 11/135 (8), p=NS	Hospital mortality: 5/100 (5)
Gustafson 1991[78]	Urinary infection: 33/103 (32.0), NS Decubital ulcers: 4/103 (3.9), p<0.05 Feeding problems: 5/103 (4.9), NS Severe falls: 0/103, p<0.05	Urinary infection: 26/111 (23.4) Decubital ulcers: 14/111 (12.6) Feeding problems: 8/111 (7.2) Severe falls: 6/111 (5.4)	Mortality rate was same in control and intervention studies	

NS=study reported finding was not significant but did not report p value; NR=not reported; AE=adverse event; CVA=cerebrovascular accident

*Other adverse events reported were anemia, constipation, depression, diarrhea, heart failure, pneumonia, other infections, myocardial infarction, pulmonary embolism, stroke, stomach ulcers, and urinary retention, and the occurrence of these was not significantly difference between intervention and control groups.

QUESTION 2a: Do these results vary by medical unit, age, gender, or comorbid conditions?

None of the included studies were stratified by medical unit, age, or comorbid conditions. Likewise, none of the studies were stratified by gender, although two studies included only men.[41,56] Therefore, we are unable to ascertain whether effectiveness varied by medical unit, age, gender or comorbid conditions.

Conclusions

Most of the included studies enrolled patients at high or very high risk of delirium as evidenced by incidence rates of delirium in the control group of 29-60%. The applicability of these findings to settings and patients with lower delirium risk is not clear. Low level evidence suggests that certain pharmacologic strategies in selected surgical settings may be useful. These include perioperative analgesia via fascia iliaca compartmental block for patients undergoing surgery for hip fracture, atypical antipsychotics, and lighter anesthesia. However, studies examining each category of prevention medications were small in size and number and inconsistencies in outcomes for various interventions occurred that are difficult to explain by patient population or setting (e.g. haloperidol was beneficial in patients undergoing gastrointestinal but not orthopedic surgery). Thus some findings could be due to chance or true effects could be missed due to small sample size and low event rates. There is low level evidence that use of cholinesterase inhibitors or perioperative statins do not reduce the risk of delirium. There is mixed evidence for continuous epidural bupivicaine plus fentanyl versus continuous IV fentanyl.

Multi-component strategies were generally successful in delirium prevention, although the interventions studied varied widely and often involved several strategies and disciplines. Thus it is difficult to determine the specific component(s) of effectiveness. Evidence suggests that staff education alone may be an effective strategy, as may be music therapy, although there are currently only two studies supporting these strategies. There is no evidence of a difference in delirium incidence associated with bright light therapy. Overall, the evidence suggests that there are few harms associated with the methods used in these studies for delirium prevention. However, it is difficult to determine the true extent of harms and whether they differ between pharmacologic and non-pharmacologic interventions due to incomplete reporting. None of the included studies were stratified by medical unit, age or comorbid conditions. Therefore, there are no data addressing whether the effectiveness or harms varies by medical unit, age, gender or comorbid conditions.

KEY QUESTION #3. What is the comparative diagnostic accuracy of the tools used to detect delirium:
a. In elderly medical and surgical inpatients?
b. In elderly ICU inpatients?

Elderly Medical and Surgical Inpatients

A recent systematic review addressed the accuracy of tools used to diagnose the presence of delirium in adults.[79] We assessed the relevance of this review as recommended in the Agency for Healthcare Research and Quality Methods Guide.[80] We found the review to be relevant - addressing the population, intervention, comparators, outcomes, timing, setting of interest for our review and including appropriate study designs. The exception was the exclusion of studies of delirium assessment for patients in an intensive care unit (ICU). We present those studies in Key Question 3b. We determined that the quality of the existing review was "good" based on the AMSTAR guidelines[81]

The review included citations from MEDLINE (1950 to May 2010), EMBASE (1980 to May 2010), and a hand-search of bibliographies of relevant articles. The review was limited to studies that included hospitalized patients (not in the ICU), used an appropriate reference standard (especially DSM-III, DSM-III-R, or DSM-IV) performed by a specialist physician, applied the same index test to more than 80% of the patients, and included patients with and without delirium. Studies that enrolled primarily children or patients with alcohol-related delirium were excluded as were studies where the same individual performed both the index and reference tests. Study quality was assessed using the method described in the Rationale Clinical Examination series as described in the Methods section.[8]

The review included 25 studies enrolling between 26 and 791 patients.[82-106] Although the review was not limited to studies of elderly patients, 15 of the 25 studies enrolled either patients older than 60 years or patients from geriatric units. In the 25 studies, 11 different diagnostic tools were used. The quality of 1 study was rated Level 1,[97] 7 were rated Level 2,[82,85,94,96,98-100] 9 were rated Level 3,[83,84,86,89,90,91,93,95,101] and 8 were rated Level 4.[87,88,92,95,103-106]

In nine studies that consecutively enrolled patients the prevalence of delirium ranged from 9% to 63%,[82,85,88,92,94,96,97,99,106] however only one study, which enrolled cancer patients consecutively referred for neurological or psychiatric consultation for mental status change, reported prevalence above 50%.[97] Five of the nine studies enrolled patients older than age 60 or from geriatric units.[82,85,88,92,96] Delirium prevalence in those studies ranged from 9% to 49%.

The most widely studied tool was the Confusion Assessment Method (CAM) with data reported from 12 studies that enrolled a total of 1036 patients[82-88,98-100,102]. CAM was developed to be administered by nonpsychiatric clinicians, is based on the 4 cardinal features of delirium, and takes approximately 5 minutes to administer.[84] There were no studies with Level of Evidence 1, 5 with Level of Evidence 2, 5 with Level of Evidence 3, and 2 with Level of Evidence 4. Sensitivity ranged from 13% to 98% with all but 2 studies greater than 75%. Specificity ranged from 77 to 100%. The pooled sensitivity was 86% and the pooled specificity was 93%. Positive test results were associated with a likelihood ratio that ranged from 4.1 to 167. The pooled likelihood ratio for a positive test was 9.6 (95%CI 5.8 to 16.0). Negative test results were associated with a likelihood ratio that ranged from 0.03 to 0.85. The pooled likelihood ratio for a negative test was 0.16 (95%CI 0.09 to 0.29). There was considerable heterogeneity in the 12 studies as reflected in I^2 values of 65% for a positive test and 85% for a negative test. In 7 studies that enrolled either patients whose age was greater than 60 years or who were identified from geriatric units, sensitivity ranged from 46% to 95% and specificity ranged from 77% to 99%. Positive likelihood ratios ranged from 4.1 to 167; negative likelihood ratios ranged from 0.05 to 0.59.

Four studies evaluated the Delirium Rating Scale (DRS), a 10-item observational scale developed to be used by clinicians with psychiatric training, and based on characteristic symptoms of delirium.[91-93,97] The studies used a value of 10 or greater (on a scale of 0 to 32) to reflect a positive test. Total enrollment in these studies was 943. The pooled sensitivity was 95% and the pooled specificity was 79%. The pooled positive and negative likelihood ratios were 4.3 (95%CI 2.1 to 9.1) and 0.07 (95%CI 0.03 to 0.37), respectively. Heterogeneity associated with the likelihood ratios was low (I^2 values of 14% and 0%, respectively). Three of the studies enrolled patients from geriatric units. Two studies used a revised version of the DRS, the DRS-R-98 (total enrollment of 129). A positive test in these studies was indicated by a score greater than 20. One of the two studies enrolled patients 65 years and older. The pooled sensitivity was 93%; pooled specificity was 89%. The positive likelihood ratio was 8.0 (95%CI 2.6 to 25, I^2 = 73%) and the negative likelihood ratio was 0.08 (95%CI 0.3 to 0.24, I^2 = 0%).

The Memorial Delirium Assessment Scale (MDAS), a 10-item clinician evaluation based on DSM criteria and requiring approximately 10 minutes to complete, was evaluated in 3 studies (a total of 330 patients).[95,101,106] One of the studies enrolled patients from a geriatric unit. A score of 10 or greater indicated a positive test. Pooled sensitivity and specificity were both 92%. The pooled positive likelihood ratio was 12 (95%CI 2.4 to 5.8, I^2 = 85%) and the pooled negative likelihood ratio was 0.9 (95%CI 0.3 to 0.38, I^2 = 69%).

Two studies reported results from assessment of the 13 item Delirium Observation Screening Scale (DOSS), a tool designed for nurses and intended to identify early symptoms of delirium as part of regular care.[89,90] The total enrollment was 178; all patients were 70 years and older. Pooled sensitivity was 92%; pooled specificity was 82%. The positive likelihood ratio was 5.2 (95%CI 2.7 to 9.9, I^2 =65%); the negative likelihood ratio was 0.10 (95%CI 0.03 to 0.37; I^2 = 0%).

Other tools identified in the review included the Clinical Assessment of Confusion (CAC), the Digit Span Test, the Global Attentiveness Rating (GAR), the Mini-Mental State Examination (MMSE), the Nursing Delirium Screening Scale (Nu-DESC), and the Vigilance "A" Test. Data were only reported from one study for each of these tools.

The study authors identified other factors that might influence the choice of a diagnostic test. A tool that can be completed in 5 minutes or less or completed by someone other than a specialist physician might be required in certain conditions.

Apart from studies examining the DRS, heterogeneity, as indicated by the I^2 values, was high. The authors explored the sources of heterogeneity in the studies that used the CAM. The I^2 associated with the negative likelihood ratio decreased from 85% to 0% when the analysis only included studies where the index text was performed by a physician. The negative likelihood ratio increased only slightly (from 0.16 to 0.19). The positive likelihood ratio increased from 9.6 to 19 but the I^2 also increased slightly (from 65% to 67%). The I^2 associated with the negative likelihood ratio also decreased to 0% when only the higher quality studies (all Level of Evidence 2) were used but the likelihood ratio again increased only slightly (from 0.16 to 0.20). The effects on the positive likelihood ratio and associated I^2 value were not reported. The authors had speculated that the version of the DSM criteria used in the study might have contributed to heterogeneity but subgroup analyses based on DSM criteria did not produce different results.

Only one of the studies included in the systematic review enrolled patients from a VA medical center[82] The focus of the study was on medical-surgical inpatients, older than age 60, who were referred to a psychiatric consultation service (PCS) for evaluation or treatment of depressive symptoms. The investigator used the CAM to assess the referred patients for delirium. A PCS psychiatrist interviewed the patients and diagnosed delirium based on DSM-III-R criteria. Only patients with concordant diagnoses by the investigator and the psychiatrist were included in the analysis (n=67). Five patients were excluded because the diagnoses were not concordant. In two cases, the psychiatrist diagnosed delirium but the investigator did not. In three cases, the investigator diagnosed delirium but the psychiatrist did not. Of the 67 patients, 28 (41.8%) were diagnosed with delirium. Twenty-four of the referrals had neither delirium nor a depressive disorder. The referring providers for 23 of the 28 delirium cases were contacted. It was determined that only 3 of the providers considered delirium in the differential diagnosis.

The authors concluded that administration of the GAR, MDAS, CAM, DRS-R-98, CAC, and DOSS all produced positive results suggestive of delirium with likelihood ratios of greater than 5.0. Similarly, normal test results that decreased the likelihood of delirium with a likelihood ratio of less than 0.2 were found in studies that used the GAR, MDAS, CAM, DRS-R-98, DRS, DOSS, Nu-DESC, and the MMSE. As noted above, some of the tools were only evaluated in one study and some studies did not focus on an elderly population. Overall, the authors recommended the use of the CAM for a time-efficient, bedside delirium assessment.

One eligible study was identified in our search of the literature published after the search dates specified in the systematic review.[107] The Level of Evidence for this study is 3. Patients (n=116) admitted to the surgical, orthopedic, or gynecological ward of one hospital were evaluated. Only elective surgery cases were included. They excluded patients who were undergoing neurosurgical procedures, or who had a history of psychiatric or neurological illness, a previous cerebral insult, or a history of drug or alcohol abuse. They also excluded patients who were unable to communicate due to severe hearing loss or brain injury. Daily delirium assessments (from preoperative day to sixth day postoperative) were performed by trained research assistants supervised by a psychiatrist. All patients were tested independently with the CAM, the Nu-DESC, and the Delirium Detection Score (DDS). Diagnosis of delirium according to DSM-IV criteria was the reference.

Of the 116 patients screened, complete data were available for 88. Although patients of any age were eligible for the study, the mean age of those with complete data was 65.5 years; 64.8% were male. Delirium was diagnosed (DSM-IV criteria) in 17 (19%). Incidence of delirium based on the other assessment tools was as follows: CAM 17%, Nu-DESC 32%, and DDS 45%. The analysis of sensitivity and specificity was based on patient days. There were a total of 512 patient days and 40 (8%) were identified as delirium according to DSM-IV criteria. With a cut-off point of 1 (greater than 1 indicating delirium), the sensitivity of the DDS was 71.2% (correct classification of 30 of the 40 patient days) and the sensitivity of the Nu-DESC was 97.7% (correct classification of 38 of 40 patient days). The overall sensitivity of the CAM was 74.9% (correct classification of 28 of 40 patient days). The CAM was the most specific (100%), followed by the Nu-DESC (92.3%), and the DDS (87.1%). The positive likelihood ratios for the CAM, Nu-DESC, and DDS were all greater than 5 while the negative likelihood ratios were all 0.33 or less.

Elderly ICU Inpatients

Instruments to detect delirium in critically ill patients, including those in the ICU, are a more recent development.[108] We identified fifteen studies, enrolling between 22 and 178 subjects, that met inclusion criteria, reporting the diagnostic accuracy of a screening/assessment tool for detection of delirium in the ICU.[109-123] Details of the studies are reported in Appendix D, Table 5.

Description of Studies

Patient Characteristics

Sample sizes ranged from 15 to 178. None of the studies reported specifically enrolling veterans. All fifteen studies reported gender, with men comprising the majority of the subjects (36 to 80%). For the thirteen studies reporting age,[109-116,118-122] the mean age ranged from 55 to 78 years. Five studies reported racial or ethnic characteristics.[109-111,115,116] Overall, the majority of the subjects in these six studies were Caucasian (50% to 88%). Six of the studies included only medical patients, six included both medical and surgical patients, one included only surgical patients, and one included only patients undergoing psychiatric care. Four of the studies included patients who were intubated;[110,112,113,118] the remainder of the studies included only patients who were not intubated. Five studies reported average ICU length of stay with values ranging from 6.0 to 9.2 days.[111,116,117,120,121]

Quality Assessment

Study quality was assessed using the method described in the Rationale Clinical Examination series as described in the Methods section.[8] Three studies were rated Level of Evidence 1,[112,113,122] four were Level 2,[114-116,123] two were Level 3,[110,111] one was Level 4,[109] and five were Level 5.[117-121]

Index and Reference Tools

In the 15 studies that met criteria, several different tools were used to identify the presence of delirium; some studies used more than one tool as the index test. The index tools studied included Confusion Assessment Method-Intensive Care Unit (CAM-ICU),[110,112,113,115,116,122] Intensive Care Delirium Screening Checklist (ICDSC),[114,117,122] Neelon and Champagne Confusion Scale (NEECHAM),[120] Delirium Detection Score (DDS),[112] CAM-ICU Flow sheet,[123] Cognitive Test for Delirium (CTD),[109] Nursing Delirium Screening Scale (Nu-DESC),[112] Memorial Delirium Assessment Scale (MDAS),[118] chart-based delirium method,[111] clinical judgment,[122] and observation checklist.[119] The index test was administered by physicians, ICU nurses, nurse researchers, trained researchers, or psychology technicians.

The reference (or "gold standard") diagnosis was determined by a psychiatrist using DSM III-R or DSM IV criteria in seven studies.[109,110,112,113,116,122,123] Another study used the DSM III-R criteria but did not report who did the assessment[119] and one study reported that the reference assessment was completed by a board certified psychiatrist but did not indicate which tool was used.[114] One study used the International Classification of Disease system (ICD-10), with the assessment by a psychiatrist, to define delirium.[118] In one study, the CAM, administered by a trained clinician researcher, was the reference test[115] while in three studies, the CAM-ICU, administered by a research nurse, was used to determine the reference diagnosis.[111,120,121] One study was a comparison of level of agreement between the ICDSC and the CAM ICU.[117]

Sensitivity and Specificity (Table 8)

The incidence of ICU delirium in the 13 studies that reported incidence ranged from 13% to 87%. It should be noted that some studies did not enroll patients consecutively. For studies using the CAM ICU and reporting sensitivity and specificity data,[110,112,113,115,116,122] sensitivity ranged from 64% to 100% and specificity ranged from 88% to 100%. One study developed a CAM-ICU Flowsheet.[123] Sensitivity and specificity averaged 90% and 100%, respectively, for two different evaluators. Sensitivity and specificity were also reported for the ICDSC (2 studies) and the Nu-DESC, DDS, CTC, MDAS, and NEECHAM (1 study each).

Other Outcomes (Table 8)

Several studies reported outcome data for patients with and without delirium. Mortality was higher for patients with delirium.[112,13,121] In one study, patients with delirium were less likely to be discharged to their home.[112] Length of stay in the ICU was higher for patients with delirium.[121,121]

Conclusions

A systematic review of bedside instruments concluded that the CAM was a suitable tool for medical and surgical inpatients, including patients in geriatric units. The conclusion was based on sensitivity, specificity, likelihood ratios and feasibility of administration. Training on use of the CAM is recommended and the tool was designed to be used during a formal cognitive assessment. Fewer studies have evaluated the diagnostic accuracy of tools to detect delirium for elderly ICU inpatients. The CAM-ICU, a version of the CAM adapted for use in the ICU, appears to have high specificity but sensitivity varies (ranging from 64 to 100%) indicating that some patients with delirium will not be identified using the CAM-ICU alone. Not all of these studies were restricted to elderly patients and most excluded patients with neurological disease or cognitive dysfunction. Other tools have been evaluated in only one or two studies.

Table 8. Outcomes – Intensive Care Unit Diagnostic Accuracy Studies

Author, Year Screening Tool	Delirium Incidence n/N (%)	Sensitivity (%)	Specificity (%)	Other Outcomes
Bergeron, 2001[114] ICDSC with cut-off score of 4	15 of 93 (16%) consecutive patients	99	64	
Ely, 2001[110] CAM-ICU	33 of 38 enrolled (87%)	Nurse 1: 95 Nurse 2: 96 Intensivist: 100	Nurse 1: 93 Nurse 2: 93 Intensivist: 89	Likelihood Ratio (+): Nurse 1: 14; Nurse 2: 14; Intensivist: 9 Accuracy 95%, 95%, 96%
Ely, 2001[116] CAM ICU	80 of 96 (83%) consecutive patients	Nurse 1: 100 Nurse 2: 93	Nurse 1: 98 Nurse 2: 100	Likelihood ratios: Nurse 1 50, Nurse 2 >100 LOS 17.9 days (mean) ICU LOS 8.3 days (mean) In hospital mortality 30.2%
Guenther, 2010[123] CAM-ICU Flowsheet	25 of 54 enrolled (46%)	Intensivist: 88 Medical Student: 92	Intensivist: 100 Medical Student: 100	
Hart, 1996[109] CTD with cut-off score <19	Not applicable	100	95	
Koolhoven, 1996[119] Observational checklist	2 of 15 enrolled (13%)	NR	NR	The 2 patients with delirium had scores >10 on DRS; 2 other patients had DRS scores >10 but symptoms did not persist so not diagnosed
Lin, 2004[113] CAM-ICU	22/102 (22%) consecutive patients	Assessor 1:91 Assessor 2: 98	Assessor 1: 95 Assessor 2: 98	Likelihood Ratio: 45.5 (Assessor 1,), 47.5 (Assessor 2) Mortality: 33% in no delirium group, 64% in delirium group
Luetz, 2010[112] CAM-ICU Nu-DESC DDS	63/156 (40%) consecutive patients	CAM-ICU: 81 Nu-DESC: 83 DDS: 30 (1st day)	CAM-ICU: 96 Nu-DESC: 81 DDS: 91 (1st day)	Mortality: 4% in no-delirium group, 24% in delirium group Discharge to home 55% in no-delirium group, 24% in delirium group
McNicoll, 2005[115] CAM ICU	11 of 22 (50%) consecutive patients	73	100	
Pisani, 2006[111] Chart-based delirium detection method	143 of 178 enrolled (80%)	64	85	All patients: ICU LOS: 8.2 days (mean); 5.0 days (median)
Plaschke, 2008[117] CAM-ICU and ICDSC	71 of 174 enrolled (41%)	N/A	N/A	Kappa coefficient .80 (CI 95%: 0.76-0.85) ICU LOS: 9.2 days (mean) Hospital LOS: 24.0 days (mean) In-hospital mortality: 19%
Shyamsundar, 2009[118] MDAS with cut-off score of 10 (unclear how many patients were assessed with reference test)	NR	100	96	

Author, Year Screening Tool	Delirium Incidence n/N (%)	Sensitivity (%)	Specificity (%)	Other Outcomes
Spronk, 2009[121] Clinical judgment	23 of 46 enrolled (50%)	Physicians: 28 Nurses 35 (for days with delirium)	Physicians: 100 Nurses: 98.3 (for days with delirium)	ICU LOS: 6 days (9 days for patients with delirium, 5 days for patients without delirium) Mortality: 24% (26% with delirium, 22% without)
van Eijk, 2009[122] CAM-ICU, ICDSC, diagnostic impression of clinician	43 of 126 enrolled (34%)	CAM-ICU: 64 ICDSC: 43 Clinician impression: 29	CAM-ICU: 88 ICDSC: 95 Clinician impression: 96	
van Rompaey, 2007[120] NEECHAM with cut-off score of <20	35 of 172 (20.3%) consecutive patients with NEECHAM, 34 of 172 (19.8%) with CAM-ICU	87	95	ICU LOS 7.0 (mean) (17.5 days for patients with delirium, 5.0 days for patients without delirium)

ICU = intensive care unit; LOS = length of stay; N/A = not applicable; NR = not reported
CAM-ICU = Confusion Assessment Method – Intensive Care Unit; CAM = Confusion Assessment Method; CTD = Cognitive Test for Delirium; DDS = Delirium Detection Score; DSM = Diagnostic and Statistical Manual of Mental Disorders; ICDSC = Intensive Care Delirium Screening Checklist; MDAS = Memorial Delirium Assessment Scale; NEECHAM = Neelon and Champagne Confusion Scale; Nu-DESC: Nursing Delirium Screening Scale

SUMMARY AND DISCUSSION

SUMMARY OF EVIDENCE BY KEY QUESTION

Key Question #1. What is the effectiveness of screening for delirium in adult inpatients?
1a. Do these results vary by medical unit, age, gender or comorbid conditions?
1b. Does screening for delirium improve clinical outcomes?

We identified no randomized controlled trials of screening for delirium in hospitalized patients. There is no direct evidence that screening for delirium is beneficial or harmful. However, universal screening may pose harms, such as misclassification, subsequent treatment of non-delirious patients or misdiagnosis of those with delirium. Opportunity costs include the time to administer screening tests and follow-up (including those of the consultants-typically a psychiatric consult) required for positive results. Additionally, we found no evidence from recent systematic reviews that pharmacologic and non-pharmacologic delirium treatments improve outcomes. Therefore, we conclude that the evidence is insufficient about the net benefit of delirium screening among all hospitalized patients or subgroups of patients as defined by age, gender, comorbidities or admission to intensive care units.

Key Question #2. What are the effectiveness and harms of delirium prevention strategies in acute elderly inpatients?
2a. Do these results vary by medical unit, age, gender or comorbid conditions?

Low level evidence suggests that pharmacologic strategies using analgesia via fascia iliaca compartmental block, antipsychotics, and lighter anesthesia may be useful in delirium prevention. However, there were only a few studies, small in size, examining each category of prevention medications, and more research is needed. Pre-operative administration of statins was not found to effect the incidence of delirium. The evidence for peri-operative use of cholinesterase inhibitors and continuous epidural bupivicaine plus fentanyl versus continuous intravenous fentanyl is mixed.

The evidence shows that multi-component strategies were generally successful in delirium prevention, although these interventions varied widely and often involved multiple strategies and disciplines, making it difficult to determine which components of the multi-component strategies may be effective. The evidence suggests that staff education alone or music therapy may be effective strategies, although there are currently only two studies supporting these interventions. There is no evidence that bright light therapy is an effective strategy for delirium prevention.

The evidence suggests that there are few harms associated with the methods used in these studies for delirium prevention. None of the included studies were stratified by medical unit, age or comorbid conditions. Therefore, we are unable to ascertain whether effectiveness or harms varied by medical unit, age, gender or comorbid conditions.

KEY QUESTION #3. What is the comparative diagnostic accuracy of the tools used to detect delirium:
3a. In elderly medical and surgical inpatients?
3b. In elderly ICU inpatients?

A systematic review of bedside instruments concluded that the CAM was a suitable tool for medical and surgical inpatients, many of whom were evaluated in geriatric units. The ease of administration (completion in less than 5 minutes) was also considered although it was noted that administrators should be trained for optimal use and that the CAM was originally developed for use in conjunction with a formal cognitive assessment. The accuracy of bedside instruments delivered by individuals without training as stand-alone tools for delirium screening is not known. Fewer studies have evaluated the diagnostic accuracy of tools to detect delirium for elderly ICU inpatients. The CAM-ICU, a version of the CAM adapted for use in the ICU, appears to have high specificity but sensitivity varies (ranging from 64 to 100%) indicating that some patients with delirium will not be identified using the CAM-ICU alone. Not all of these studies were restricted to elderly patients and most excluded patients with neurological disease or cognitive dysfunction. Other tools have been evaluated in only one or two studies.

RECOMMENDATIONS FOR FUTURE RESEARCH

The highest future research need is to conduct a randomized trial to evaluate the effectiveness and harms of screening for delirium in adults admitted to hospitals. Enrollment could target individuals likely to be at increased risk for, and thus hopefully at greatest benefit of, successful screening, prevention and treatment options. These could include individuals who are elderly, those with multiple comorbid conditions including mental health and cognitive impairment, and those receiving or likely to receive interventions or medications that can increase the risk of delirium and patients admitted to intensive care units. Additional work is needed to more clearly assess the harms associated with delirium screening and prevention, including the opportunity costs to health service personnel. These opportunity costs include the time and effort to administer screening tools as well as the downstream effects that occur based on follow-up of positive screen results or the efforts required for preventive strategies. More research is needed to verify the findings that some pharmacologic and non-pharmacologic strategies are helpful in the prevention of delirium, particularly in larger and more diverse populations, and with reports stratified by age, medical unit and comorbid conditions. Additionally, more research is needed to start to identify which components of the multi-component non-pharmacologic strategies may be most successful in delirium prevention. Investigations regarding delirium that may be provoked only by certain medication use (in the absence of other causes) would be very helpful; they may well have different prognoses than the multifactorial delirium. This research may offer some recommendations for prevention strategies that could easily be implemented. Finally, continued evaluation of diagnostic tools is warranted including the effects of training on diagnostic accuracy and the use of the tools in combination with other (e.g., cognitive) patient assessments.

CONCLUSIONS

Our review of the evidence on screening for and prevention and diagnosis of delirium finds the following:

1. There is insufficient evidence regarding benefits and harms of delirium screening in hospitalized patients including subgroups of patients as defined by age, gender, comorbidities, or ICU admission. We identified no randomized trials of screening for delirium in hospitalized patients. Conducting large pragmatic delirium screening trials is a high-priority research need.

2. There are low quality data regarding pharmacological strategies to prevent delirium. Many proactive preventive strategies have not been examined; those that have are typically reported in only a single trial. In addition, sample sizes are typically small, populations represent only selected groups of patients, and there is little consistency or completeness of outcomes reporting.

3. Multi-component interventions hold promise and are widely used in real world settings but few randomized trials have been reported. The absolute effectiveness and the contributing effectiveness of individual components is not well known but most appear to include some method of staff education to increase awareness of signs/symptoms and encourage reporting of delirium with subsequent earlier intervention.

4. Available diagnostic tests have acceptable diagnostic operating characteristics in the populations and settings where they have been studied and when administered by individuals with adequate training. Concurrent mental status testing may also be a factor in accuracy of diagnosis with these tests. It is not known whether the operating characteristics are robust across a wide range of populations and settings where the prevalence and incidence of delirium varied from the reported studies.

5. Additional research is needed to evaluate the clinical effectiveness and harms of screening, pharmacological and non-pharmacological interventions to prevent delirium applied to a larger and more diverse population, and diagnostic tools used in a broader range of populations and settings.

REFERENCES

1. Cole MG, Ciampi A, Belzile E, Zhong L. Persistent delirium in older hospital patients: a systematic review of frequency and prognosis. *Age Ageing.* 2009;38:19-26.

2. Witlox J, Eurelings LS, de Jonghe JF, Kalisvaart KJ, Eikelenboom P, van Gool WA. Delirium in elderly patients and the risk of postdischarge mortality, institutionalization, and dementia: a meta-analysis. *JAMA.* 2010;304:443-51.

3. Marcantonio ER. In the Clinic: Delirium. *Ann Intern Med.* 2011;154:ITC6-1-ITC6-16.

4. Rudolph JS, Marcantonaio ER. Postoperative delirium: acute change with long-term implications. *Anesth Analg.* 2011;112:1202-11.

5. Inouye SK, Foreman MD, Mion LC, Katz KH, Cooney LM. Nurses' recognition of delirum and its symptoms. Comparison of nurse and researcher ratings. *Arch Intern Med.* 2001;161:2467-73.

6. Inouye SK. Delirium in older persons. *N Engl J Med.* 2006;354:1157-65.

7. Delirium: diagnosis, prevention and management. Revision July 2010. Available at www.nice.org.uk/CG103. Accessed March 30, 2011.

8. Simel DL. Update: primer on precision and accuracy. In: Simel DL, Rennie D, eds. *Rationale Clinical Examination: The Evidence-Based Clinical Diagnosis.* New York, NY: McGraw-Hill; 2009:9-16.

9. Levkoff S, Cleary P, Liptzin B, Evans DA. Epidemiology of delirium: an overview of research issues and findings. *Int Psychogeriatr.* 1991;3:149-67.

10. Trzepacz PT. Delirium. Advances in diagnosis, pathophysiology, and treatment. *Psychiatr Clin North Am.* 1996;19:429-48.

11. Francis J, Martin D, Kapoor WN. A prospective study of delirium in hospitalized elderly. *JAMA.* 1990;263:1097-101.

12. Dautzenberg PLJ, Mulder LJ, Olde Rikkert MGM, Wouters CJ, Loonen AJM. Delirium in elderly hospitalised patients: protective effects of chronic rivastigmine usage. *Int J Geriatr Psychiatry.* 2004;19:641-4.

13. Williams-Russo P, Urquhart BL, Sharrock NE, Charlson ME. Post-operative delirium: predictors and prognosis in elderly orthopedic patients. *J Am Geriatr Soc.* 1992;40:759-67.

14. McCusker J, Cole M, Abrahamowicz M, Primeau F, Belzile E. Delirium predicts 12-month mortality. *Arch Intern Med.* 2002;162:457-63.

15. Inouye SK, Rushing JT, Foreman MD, Palmer RM, Pompei P. Does delirium contribute to poor hospital outcomes? A three-site epidemiologic study. *J Gen Intern Med.* 1998;13:234-42.

16.   Stevens LE, de Moore GM, Simpson JM. Delirium in hospital: does it increase length of stay? *Aust N Z J Psychiatry.* 1998;32:805-8.

17.   Inouye SK. The dilemma of delirium: clinical and research controversies regarding diagnosis and evaluation of delirium in hospitalized elderly medical patients. *Am J Med.* 1994;97:278-88.

18.   Lemiengre J, Nellis T, Joosten E, et al. Detection of delirium by bedside nurses using the confusion assessment method. *J Am Geriatr Soc.* 2006;54:685-9.

19.   Higgins JPT, Green S (eds). *Cochrane Handbook for Systematic Reviews of Interventions.* Version 5.0.2 [updated September 2009]. The Cochrane Collaboration, 2009. Available at www.cochrane-handbook.org. Accessed August 29, 2011.

20.   Owens DK, Lohr KN, Atkins D, et al. AHRQ series paper 5: grading the strength of a body of evidence when comparing medical interventions--agency for healthcare research and quality and the effective health-care program. *J Clin Epidemiol.* 2010;63:513-23.

21.   Siddiqi N, Stockdale R, Britton AM, Holmes J. Interventions for preventing delirium in hospitalised patients. Cochrane Database Syst Rev 2007:CD005563.

22.   O'Mahoney R, Murthy L, Akunne A, Young J, for the Guideline Development Group. Synopsis of the National Institute for Health and Clinical Excellence guideline for prevention of delirium. *Ann Intern Med.* 2011;154:746-51.

23.   Diaz V, Rodriguez J, Barrientos P, et al. [Use of procholinergics in the prevention of post-operative delirium in hip fracture surgery in the elderly. A randomized controlled trial]. *Rev Neurol* 2001;33:716-9.

24.   Hennekens CH, Buring JE, Mayrent SL. *Epidemiology in medicine.* Chicago, IL: Lippincott Williams & Wilkins; 1987.

25.   *Clinical Practice Guidelines for the Management of Delirium in Older People.* Revision October 2006. Available at www.health.vic.gov.au/acute-agedcare/delirium-cpg.pdf. Accessed March 30, 2011.

26.   Siddiqi N, House AO, Holmes JD. Occurrence and outcome of delirium in medical in-patients: a systematic literature review. *Age Ageing.* 2006;35:350-64.

27.   Lonergan E, Britton AM, Luxenberg J, Wyller T. Antipsychotics for delirium. Cochrane Database Syst Rev 2007:CD005594.

28.   Seitz DP, Gill SS, van Zyl LT. Antipsychotics in the treatment of delirium: a systematic review. *J Clin Psychiatry.* 2007;68:11-21.

29.   Campbell N, Boustani MA, Ayub A, et al. Pharmacological management of delirium in hospitalized adults--a systematic evidence review. *J Gen Intern Med.* 2009;24:848-53.

30.   Fong TG, Tulebaev SR, Inouye SK. Delirium in elderly adults: diagnosis, prevention and treatment. *Nat Rev Neurol.* 2009;5:210-20.

31.   Young J, Murthy L, Westby M, Akunne A, O'Mahony R. Diagnosis, prevention, and management of delirium: summary of NICE guidance. *BMJ.* 2010;341:247-9.

32.   Michaud L, Bula C, Berney A, et al. Delirium: guidelines for general hospitals. *J Psychosom Res.* 2007;62:371-83.

33.   *Guidelines for the prevention, diagnosis and management of delirium in older people in hospital.* Revision January 2006. Available at http://www.bgs.org.uk/Publications/Clinical%20Guidelines/clinical_1-2_delirium.htm. Accessed March 30, 2011.

34.   Jacobi J, Fraser GL, Coursin DB, et al. Clinical practice guidelines for the sustained use of sedatives and analgesics in the critically ill adult. *Crit Care Med.* 2002;30:119-41.

35.   Wei LA, Fearing MA, Sternberg EJ, Inouye SK. The Confusion Assessment Method: a systematic review of current usage. *J Am Geriatr Soc.* 2008;56:823-30.

36.   *Delirium.* Revision April 24, 2010: Available at http://www.mayoclinic.com/health/delirium/DS01064. Accessed August 11, 2011.

37.   Al-Aama T, Brymer C, Gutmanis I, Woolmore-Goodwin SM, Esbaugh J, Dasgupta M. Melatonin decreases delirium in elderly patients: a randomized, placebo-controlled trial. *Int J Geriatr Psychiatry* 2011;26:687-94.

38.   Larsen KA, Kelly SE, Stern TA, et al. Administration of olanzapine to prevent postoperative delirium in elderly joint-replacement patients: A randomized, controlled trial. *Psychosomatics.* 2010;51:409-18.

39.   Sieber FE, Zakriya KJ, Gottschalk A, et al. Sedation depth during spinal anesthesia and the development of postoperative delirium in elderly patients undergoing hip fracture repair. *Mayo Clin Proc.* 2010;85:18-26.

40.   Gamberini M, Bolliger D, Lurati Buse GA, et al. Rivastigmine for the prevention of postoperative delirium in elderly patients undergoing elective cardiac surgery--a randomized controlled trial. *Crit Care Med.* 2009;37:1762-8.

41.   Hudetz JA, Patterson KM, Iqbal Z, et al. Ketamine attenuates delirium after cardiac surgery with cardiopulmonary bypass. *J Cardiothorac Vasc Anesth.* 2009;23:651-7.

42.   Maldonaldo JR, Wysong A, van der Staare PJA, Block T, Miller C, Reitz BA. Dexmedetomidine and the reduction of postoperative delirium after cardiac surgery. *Psychosomatics.* 2009;50:206-17.

43.   Mouzopoulos G, Vasiliadis G, Lasanianos N, Nikolaras G, Morakis E, Kaminaris M. Fascia iliaca block prophylaxis for hip fracture patients at risk for delirium: a randomized placebo-controlled study. *J Orthop Traumatol.* 2009;10:127-33.

44.   Prakanrattana U, Prapaitrakool S. Efficacy of risperidone for prevention of postoperative delirium in cardiac surgery. *Anaesth Intensive Care.* 2007;35:714-9.

45.   Sampson EL, Raven PR, Ndhlovu PN, et al. A randomized, double-blind, placebo-controlled trial of donepezil hydrochloride (Aricept) for reducing the incidence of postoperative delirium after elective total hip replacement. *Int J Geriatr Psychiatry.* 2007;22:343-9.

46.   Kalisvaart KJ, de Jonghe JF, Bogaards MJ, et al. Haloperidol prophylaxis for elderly hip-surgery patients at risk for delirium: a randomized placebo-controlled study. *J Am Geriatr Soc.* 2005;53:1658-66.

47.   Liptzin B, Laki A, Garb JL, Fingeroth R, Krushell R. Donepezil in the prevention and treatment of post-surgical delirium. *Am J Geriatr Psychiatry.* 2005;13:1100-6.

48.   Papaioannou A, Fraidakis O, Michaloudis D, Balalis C, Askitopoulou H. The impact of the type of anesthesia on cognitive status and delirium during the first postoperative days in elderly patients. *Eur J Anaesthesiol.* 2005;22:492-9.

49.   Aizawa K, Kanai T, Saikawa Y, et al. A novel approach to the prevention of postoperative delirium in the elderly after gastrointestinal surgery. *Surg Today.* 2002;32:310-4.

50.   Kaneko T, Cai J, Ishikura T, et al. Prophylactic consecutive administration of haloperidol can reduce the occurrence of postoperative delirium in gastrointestinal surgery. *Yonago Acta Medica.* 1999.42:179-84.

51.   Berggren D, Gustafson Y, Eriksson B, et al. Postoperative confusion after anesthesia in elderly patients with femoral neck fractures. *Anesth Analg.* 1987;66:497-504.

52.   Katznelson R, Djaiani GN, Borger MA, et al. Preoperative use of statins is associated with reduced early delirium rates after cardiac surgery. *Anesthesiology.* 2009;110:67-73.

53.   Del Rosario E, Esteve N, Sernandez MJ, Batet C, Aguilar JL. Does femoral nerve analgesia impact the development of postoperative delirium in the elderly? A retrospective investigation. *Acute Pain.* 2008;10:59-64.

54.   Savage GJ, Metzger JT. The prevention of postanesthetic delirium. *Plast Reconstr Surg.* 1978;62:81-4.

55.   Lundstrom M, Olofsson B, Stenvall M, et al. Postoperative delirium in old patients with femoral neck fracture: a randomized intervention study. *Aging Clin Exp Res.* 2007;19:178-86.

56.   Taguchi T, Yano M, Kido Y. Influence of bright light therapy on postoperative patients: a pilot study. *Intensive Crit Care Nurs.* 2007;23:289-97.

57.   McCaffrey R, Locsin R. The effect of music on pain and acute confusion in older adults undergoing hip and knee surgery. *Holist Nurs Pract.* 2006;20:218-26.

58.   Lundstrom M, Edlund A, Karlsson S, Brunnstrom B, Bucht G, Gustafson Y. A multifactorial intervention program reduces the duration of delirium, length of hospitalization, and mortality in delirious patients. *J Am Geriatr Soc.* 2005;53:622-8.

59.   Marcantonio ER, Flacker JM, Wright RJ, Resnick NM. Reducing delirium after hip frac-
       ture: a randomized trial. *J Am Geriatr Soc.* 2001;49:516-22.

60.   Ushida T, Yokoyama T, Kishida Y, et al. Incidence and risk factors of postoperative de-
       lirium in cervical spine surgery. *Spine.* 2009;34:2500-4.

61.   Vidan M, T., Sanchez E, Alonso M, Montero B, Ortiz J, Serra J. An intervention inte-
       grated into daily clinical practice reduces the incidence of delirium during hospitalization
       in elderly patients. *J Am Geriatr Soc.* 2009;57:2029-36.

62.   Kratz A. Use of the acute confusion protocol: a research utilization project. *J Nurs Care
       Qual.* 2008;23:331-7.

63.   Robinson S, Rich C, Weitzel T, Vollmer C, Eden B. Delirium prevention for cognitive,
       sensory, and mobility impairments. *Res Theory Nurs Pract.* 2008;22:103-13.

64.   Vollmer C, Rich C, Robinson S. How to prevent delirium: a practical protocol. *Nursing.*
       2007;37:26-8.

65.   Caplan GA, Harper EL. Recruitment of volunteers to improve vitality in the elderly: the
       REVIVE study. *Intern Med J.* 2007;37:95-100.

66.   Harari D, Hopper A, Dhesi J, Babic-Illman G, Lockwood L, Martin F. Proactive care of
       older people undergoing surgery ('POPS'): designing, embedding, evaluating and fund-
       ing a comprehensive geriatric assessment service for older elective surgical patients. *Age
       Ageing.* 2007;36:190-6.

67.   Naughton BJ, Saltzman S, Ramadan F, Chadha N, Priore R, Mylotte JM. A multifactorial
       intervention to reduce prevalence of delirium and shorten hospital length of stay. *J Am
       Geriatr Soc.* 2005;53:18-23.

68.   Tabet N, Hudson S, Sweeney V, et al. An educational intervention can prevent delirium
       on acute medical wards. *Age Ageing.* 2005;34:152-6.

69.   Wong DM, Niam T, Bruce JJ, Bruce DG. Quality project to prevent delirium after hip
       fracture. *Australasian J Ageing.* 2005;24:174-7.

70.   Milisen K, Foreman MD, Abraham IL, et al. A nurse-led interdisciplinary intervention
       program for delirium in elderly hip-fracture patients. *J Am Geriatr Soc.* 2001;49:523-32.

71.   Inouye SK, Bogardus ST, Jr., Charpentier PA, et al. A multicomponent intervention to
       prevent delirium in hospitalized older patients. *N Engl J Med.* 1999;340:669-76.

72.   Rizzo JA, Bogardus ST, Jr., Leo-Summers L, Williams CS, Acampora D, Inouye SK.
       Multicomponent targeted intervention to prevent delirium in hospitalized older patients:
       what is the economic value? *Med Care.* 2001;39:740-52.

73.   Inouye SK, Bogardus ST, Jr., Williams CS, Leo-Summers L, Agostini JV. The role of
       adherence on the effectiveness of nonpharmacologic interventions: evidence from the
       delirium prevention trial. *Arch Intern Med.* 2003;163:958-64.

74.   Leslie DL, Zhang Y, Bogardus ST, Holford TR, Leo-Summers LS, Inouye SK. Conse-
       quences of preventing delirium in hospitalized older adults on nursing home costs. *J Am
       Geriatr Soc.* 2005;53:405-9.

75.   Leslie DL, Zhang Y, Holford TR, Bogardus ST, Leo-Summers LS, Inouye SK. Premature
       death associated with delirium at 1-year follow-up. *Arch Intern Med.* 2005;165:1657-62.

76.   Lundstrom M, Edlund A, Lundstrom G, Gustafson Y. Reorganization of nursing and
       medical care to reduce the incidence of postoperative delirium and improve rehabilita-
       tion outcome in elderly patients treated for femoral neck fractures. *Scand J Caring Sci.*
       1999;13:193-200.

77.   Wanich CK, Sullivan-Marx EM, Gottlieb GL, Johnson JC. Functional status outcomes of
       a nursing intervention in hospitalized elderly. *Image J Nurs Sch.* 1992;24(3):201-7.

78.   Gustafson Y, Brännström B, Berggren D, et al. A geriatric-anesthesiologic program to
       reduce acute confusional states in elderly patients treated for femoral neck fractures. *J
       Am Geriatric Soc.* 1991;39:655-62.

79.   Wong CL, Holroyd-Leduc J, Simel DL, Straus SE. Does this patient have delirium?:
       value of bedside instruments. *JAMA.* 2010;304:779-86.

80.   White CM, Ip S, McPheeters M, et al. Using Existing Systematic Reviews To Replace De
       Novo Processes in Conducting Comparative Effectiveness Reviews. In: *Methods Guide
       for Comparative Effectiveness Reviews.* 2011/03/25 ed. Rockville, MD: Agency for
       Healthcare Research and Quality; 2008.

81.   Shea BJ, Grimshaw JM, Wells GA, et al. Development of AMSTAR: a measurement tool
       to assess the methodological quality of systematic reviews. *BMC Med Res Methodol.*
       2007;7:10.

82.   Farrell KR, Ganzini L. Misdiagnosing delirium as depression in medically ill elderly
       patients. *Arch Intern Med.* 1995;155:2459-64.

83.   González M, de Pablo J, Fuente E, et al. Instrument for detection of delirium in general
       hospitals: adaptation of the confusion assessment method. *Psychosomatics.* 2004;45:426-
       31.

84.   Inouye SK, van Dyck CH, Alessi CA, Balkin S, Siegal AP, Horwitz RI. Clarifying confu-
       sion: the confusion assessment method. A new method for detection of delirium. *Ann
       Intern Med.* 1990;113:941-8.

85.   Laurila JV, Pitkala KH, Strandberg TE, Tilvis RS. Confusion Assessment Method in the
       diagnostics of delirium among aged hospital patients: Would it serve better in screening
       than as a diagnostic instrument? *Int J Geriatr Psychiatry.* 2002;17:1112-9.

86. Leung JM, Leung VW, Leung CM, Pan PC. Clinical utility and validation of two instruments (the Confusion Assessment Method algorithm and the Chinese version of Nursing Delirium Screening Scale) to detect delirium in geriatric inpatients. *Gen Hosp Psychiatry.* 2008;30:171-6.

87. Pompei P, Foreman M, Cassel C, Alessi C, Cox D. Detecting delirium among hospitalized older patients. *Arch Intern Med.* 1995;155:301-7.

88. Zou Y, Cole MJ, Rimeau FJ, McCusker J, Bellavance F. Laplante J. Detection and diagnosis of delirium in the elderly: psychiatrist diagnosis, Confusion Assessment Method, or consensus diagnosis? *Int Psychogeriatr.* 1998;10:303-8.

89. Gemert van LA, Schuurmans MJ. The Neecham Confusion Scale and the Delirium Observation Screening Scale: Capacity to discriminate and ease of use in clinical practice. *BMC Nursing.* 2007,6:3.

90. Schuurmans MJ, Shortridge-Bagget LM, Duursma SA. The Delirium Observation Screening Scale: a screening instrument for delirium. *Res Theory Nurs Pract.* 2003;17:31-50.

91. Rockwood K, Goodman J, Flynn M, Stolee P. Cross-validation of the Delirium Rating Scale in older patients. *J Am Geriatr* Soc 1996;44:839-42.

92. Rosen J, Sweet RA, Mulsant BH, Rifai AH, Pasternak R, Zubenko GS. The Delirium Rating Scale in a psychogeriatric inpatient setting. *J Neuropsychiatry Clin Neurosci.* 1994;6:30-5.

93. Trzepacz PT, Brenner RP, Coffman G, van Thiel DH. Delirium in liver transplantation candidates. *Biol Psychiatry.* 1988;24:3-14.

94. de Rooij SE, van Munster BC, Korevaar JC, et al. Delirium subtype identification and the validation of the Delirium Rating Scale-Revised-98 (Dutch version) in hospitalized elderly patients. *Int J Geriatr Psychiatry.* 2006;21:876-82.

95. Matsouka Y, Miyake Y, Arakaki H, Tanaka K, Saeki T, Yamawaki S. Clinical utility and validation of the Japanese version of Memorial Delirium Assessment Scale in a psychogeriatric inpatient setting. *Gen Hosp Psychiatry.* 2001;23:36-40.

96. O'Keeffe ST, Gosney MA. Assessing attentiveness in older hospital patients: global assessment versus tests of attention. *J Am Geriatr Soc.* 1997;45:470-3.

97. Grassi L, Caraceni A, Beltrami E, et al. Assessing delirium in cancer patients. The Italian versions of the Delirium Rating Scale and the Memorial Delirium Assessment Scale. *J Pain Symptom Manage.* 2001;21:59-68.

98. Hestermann U, Bakenstrass M, Gekle I, et al. Validation of a German version of the Confusion Assessment Method for delirium detection in a sample of acute geriatric patients with a high prevalence of dementia. *Psychopathology.* 2009;42:270-6.

99. Rolfson DB, McElhaney JE, Jhangri GS, Rockwood K. Validity of the confusion assessment method in detecting postoperative delirium in the elderly. *Int Psychogeriatr.* 1999;11:431-8.

100. Ryan K, Leonard M, Guerin S, Donnelly S, Conroy M, Meagher D. Validation of the Confusion Assessment Method in the palliative care setting. *Palliat Med.* 2009;23:40-5.

101. Breitbart W, Rosenfeld B, Roth A, Smith MJ, Cohen K, Passik S. The Memorial Delirium Assessment Scale. *J Pain Symptom Manage.* 1997;13:128-37.

102. Gaudreau JD, Gagnosn P, Harel F, Roy MA. Impact on delirium detection of using a sensitive instrument integrated into clinical practice. *Gen Hosp Psychiatry.* 2005;27:194-9.

103. Andrew MK, Bhat R, Clark B, Freter SH, Rockwood MRH, Rockwood K. Inter-rater reliability of the DRS-R-98 in detecting delirium in frail elderly patients. *Age Ageing.* 2009;28(2):241-4.

104. de Negreiros DP, da Silva Meleiro AMA, Furlanetto LM, Trzepacz PT. Portuguese version of the Delirium Rating Scale-Revised-98: reliability and validity. *Int J Geriatr Psychiatry.* 2008;23:472-7.

105. Huang MC, Lee CH, Lai YC, Kao YF, Lin HY, Chen CH. Chinese version of the Delirium Rating Scale-Revised-98: reliability and validity. *Compr Psychiatry.* 2009;50:81-5.

106. Kazmierski J, Kowman M, Banach M, et al. Clinical utility and use of DSM-IV and ICD-10 criteria and the Memorial Delirium Assessment Scale in establishing a diagnosis of delirium after cardiac surgery. *Psychosomatics.* 2008;49:73-6.

107. Radtke FM, Franck M, Schust S, et al. A comparison of three scores to screen for delirium on the surgical ward. *World J Surg.* 2010;34:487-94.

108. Bruno JJ, Warren ML. Intensive care unit delirium. *Crit Care Nurs Clin North Am.* 2010;22:161-78.

109. Hart RP, Levenson JL, Sessler CN, Best AM, Schwartz SM, Rutherford LE. Validation of a cognitive test for delirium in medical ICU patients. *Psychosomatics.* 1996;37:533-46.

110. Ely EW, Margolin R, Francis J, et al. Evaluation of delirium in critically ill patients: validation of the Confusion Assessment Method for the Intensive Care Unit (CAM-ICU). *Crit Care Med.* 2001;29:1370-9.

111. Pisani MA, Araujo KLB, Van Ness PH, Zhang Y, Ely EW, Inouye SK. A research algorithm to improve detection of delirium in the intensive care unit. *Crit Care.* 2006;10:R121.

112. Luetz A, Heymann A, Radtke FM, et al. Different assessment tools for intensive care unit delirium: which score to use? *Crit Care Med.* 2010;38:409-18.

113. Lin S-M, Liu C-Y, Wang C-H, et al. The impact of delirium on the survival of mechanically ventilated patients. *Crit Care Med.* 2004;32:2254-9.

114. Bergeron N, Dubois MJ, Dumont M, Dial S, Skrobik Y. Intensive Care Delirium Screening Checklist: evaluation of a new screening tool. *Intensive Care Med.* 2001;27:859-64.

115. McNicoll L, Pisani MA, Ely EW, Gifford D, Inouye SK. Detection of delirium in the intensive care unit: comparison of confusion assessment method for the intensive care unit with confusion assessment method ratings. *J Am Geriatr Soc.* 2005;53:495-500.

116. Ely EW, Inouye SK, Bernard GR, et al. Delirium in mechanically ventilated patients: validity and reliability of the confusion assessment method for the intensive care unit (CAM-ICU). *JAMA.* 2001;286:2703-10.

117. Plaschke K, von Haken R, Scholz M, et al. Comparison of the confusion assessment method for the intensive care unit (CAM-ICU) with the Intensive Care Delirium Screening Checklist (ICDSC) for delirium in critical care patients gives high agreement rate(s). *Intensive Care Med.* 2008;34:431-6.

118. Shyamsundar G, Raghuthaman G, Rajkumar AP, Jacob KS. Validation of memorial delirium assessment scale. *J Crit Care.* 2009;24:530-4.

119. Koolhoven I, Tjon-A-Tsien MR, van der Mast RC. Early diagnosis of delirium after cardiac surgery. *Gen Hosp Psychiatry.* 1996;18:448-51.

120. Van Rompaey B, Schuurmans MJ, Shortridge-Baggett LM, Truijen S, Elseviers M, Bossaert L. A comparison of the CAM-ICU and the NEECHAM Confusion Scale in intensive care delirium assessment: an observational study in non-intubated patients. *Crit Care.* 2008;12:R16.

121. Spronk PE, Riekerk B, Hofhuis J, Rommes JH. Occurrence of delirium is severely underestimated in the ICU during daily care. *Intensive Care Med.* 2009;35:1276-80.

122. van Eijk MMJ, van Marum RJ, Klijn IAM, de Wit N, Kesecioglu J, Slooter AJC. Comparison of delirium assessment tools in a mixed intensive care unit. *Crit Care Med.* 2009;37:1881-5.

123. Guenther U, Popp J, Koecher L, et al. Validity and reliability of the CAM-ICU Flowsheet to diagnose delirium in surgical ICU patients. *J Crit Care.* 2010;25:144-51.

APPENDIX A. SEARCH STRATEGIES

Delirium screening and diagnosis

Database: Ovid MEDLINE(R)
Search Strategy:

1	confusion.mp. or exp Confusion/
2	exp Delirium/ or delirium.mp.
3	deliri$.tw.
4	(NEECHAM or "Neelon and Champagne Confusion Scale").tw.
5	(MMSE or mini-mental stat$ exam$).tw.
6	or/1-5
7	sensitiv$.mp.
8	predictive value$.mp.
9	accurac$.tw.
10	or/7-9
11	6 and 10
12	limit 11 to english language
13	mass screening.mp. or exp Mass Screening/
14	diagnosis.mp. or exp Diagnosis/
15	13 or 14
16	12 and 15

Delirium prevention

Database: Ovid MEDLINE(R) <1950 to November Week 2 2010>
Search Strategy:

1	exp Delirium/
2	deliri*.mp.
3	exp Confusion/ or acute confusion.mp.
4	acute organic psychosyndrome.mp.
5	acute brain syndrome.mp.
6	metabolic encephalopathy.mp.
7	acute psycho-organic syndrome.mp.
8	clouded state.mp.
9	clouding of consciousness.mp.
10	exogenous psychosis.mp.
11	toxic psychosis.mp.
12	toxic confusion.mp.
13	or/1-12
14	exp Primary Prevention/
15	prevent*.mp.
16	avoid*.mp.
17	or/14-16

18   13 and 17
19   exp Alcohol Withdrawal Delirium/
20   delirium tremens.ti.
21   19 or 20
22   18 not 21
23   exp animals/ not humans.sh.
24   22 not 23
25   limit 24 to english language
26   limit 25 to yr="1966 -Current"

APPENDIX B. STUDY SELECTION FORM

First Author	Eligible Study? Y N	If N, what # below? 1 2 3 4 5 6 7 8 9 10 11

	Screening? Y N	Prevention? Y N	Diagnosis? Y N

Title of Study	Journal	Country	Year

Study Design	Cohort	Cross-sectional	Case-control	RCT	Non-RCT	Review/Meta-analysis

Sample	Sample size	Inclusion Criteria	Exclusion Criteria
	Veteran? Y N	Elderly 60+? Y N	ICU? Y N
	Gender? M F	Age Range?	Ethnicity?

Screening, Diagnostic Tools or Approaches Used:

CAM	CAM-ICU	MMSE	ICDSC	DRS	MDAS	DSM-IV	Others/Details:

Prevention strategies:
- Nursing interventions
- Hydration
- Music
- Medications

Findings/Outcomes:

Diagnostic accuracy	Delirium incidence	Delirium duration/severity	Length of stay	Use of rescue meds	Discharge to rehab/NH	Health economics	Others/Details:

Exclusion Criteria (*=does not apply to Prevention Studies)

1	2	3	4	5*	6*	7*	8	9	10	11
Non-English	<16 yo	Alcohol-related	Not hospitalized	No reference standard	Reference standard not done by specialist	Same person did test/reference standard	Case series/ report, letter, or editorial	Not delirium	No outcomes of interest	Not screening, prevention, diagnosis

APPENDIX C. PEER REVIEW COMMENTS/AUTHOR RESPONSES

REVIEWER COMMENT	RESPONSE
1. Are the objectives, scope, and methods for this review clearly described?	
Yes. The incidence of delirium is a significant complication of hospitalization that warrants further review. The ability for identification and prevention of delirium in medically ill patients is a current need. The objectives of this study were clearly stated and it appears that a large data base of research was examined to address the key questions posed by this review.	
Yes	
Yes	
Yes. I think Key Question #1 includes multiple disparate elements "effectiveness" is really answered by question #3 diagnostic accuracy, as is vary in results. In the summary, only does screening improve clinical outcomes is answered.	Effectiveness is not adequately addressed by KQ3 "diagnostic accuracy". While there was no direct evidence of the effectiveness and harms of screening for delirium we have described in the KQ1 results section the pieces of chain of evidence that would need to be addressed for indirect evidence of effectiveness.
Yes	
2. Is there any indication of bias in our synthesis of the evidence?	
No.	
No	
No	
No	
No. Honestly, I have a sense of bias, but it is hard to identify the source. I am a little worried that your questions are so narrow that a naïve reader will say… well, there is nothing new here since 1970. When in fact, it is pretty clear that delirium is associated with mortality, that some drugs are used more commonly in patients who develop delirium, that haldol can attenuate the consequences of delirium, that benzodiazepines in patients at risk should be avoided……….	The scope of this report was not to assess all pharmacologic interventions that increase a person's risk of delirium. However, we have added categories of medications widely recognized to be associated with delirium. We also have described that delirium is associated with mortality.
No	
3. Are there any published or underlined or unpublished studies that we may have overlooked?	
No. Not to my knowledge.	
No. This is an amazing compendium of information, and I have little to add, especially given comment about authors' awareness of, and plans to include information from, June 2011 article in Annals of Internal Medicine.	Thank you
No	
There are pending publications from 2 studies (Boustani and Marcantonio) on cholinesterase inhibitors and their role in delirium prevention.	Our inclusion criteria required articles be published in peer review manuscripts.
I don't know the literature sufficiently to know.	
I am not aware of any studies that were overlooked.	

REVIEWER COMMENT	RESPONSE
4. Are there any clinical performance measures, programs, quality improvement measures, patient care services, or conferences that will be directly affected by this report? If so, please provide detail.	Thank you – we will share these suggestions with the people responsible for dissemination of the report.
Presently OQP reviews inpatient records for evidence of elevated risk for delirium. Because these efforts are still in a relatively early stage, not much attention has been drawn to them—but as the data and the outcome correlations become more robust, educational efforts can be undertaken to support use of the QI and thereby, to enhance quality of inpt. care. Some of these data were presented at a recent VA conference (EES) in Indianapolis that focused on safety enhancement in different health delivery settings. In the two preceding years (2009, 2010), national conferences concerning delirium prevention, recognition, and management were also held in Boston and Baltimore. Plans are just beginning for a "Emergency Rooms and the Elderly Veteran" conference for Spring 2012. OQP is also examining a proposal from GEC to adapt a number of the "Assessing Care of Vulnerable Elderly" QIs to VA—several of these have to do with documenting mental status upon hospital admission in order to have a baseline against which subsequent mental status may be compared.
The Office of Geriatrics and Extended Care currently supports several demonstration pilots (about to embark on their 3rd years of funding) specifically directed to delirium prevention in different settings: in San Francisco, an Acute Care for the Elderly unit; in Connecticut, a home-based presurgical assessment followed by post-discharge transition management; in Boston, a "Delirium Toolbox" for reducing risk factors in recent admissions with demonstrated elevated risk for delirium; in Durham, a caregiver education program to assist with behaviors associated with cognitive decline; in Indianapolis, a transition management approach that begins during an inpatient stay; and in New Orleans, Portland, Boise, and Honolulu, a "Hospital at Home" that provides an inpatient level of care in the home for targeted diagnoses, with complete avoidance of delirium.
There is a national Dementia Steering Committee that developed a strategic plan and has educational, clinical, and research activities underway. Because dementia is one of the most concerning risk factors for delirium onset, this group's awareness of this information will unquestionably be of interest.
The final report of the USH-chartered "Healthcare Workforce for Aging Veterans" Executive Taskforce has been the subject of three briefings with Dr. Petzel and, with his approval, is about to be presented to the National Leadership Board—it recommends focusing resources over the next 5 years on ensuring universal access within VHA to a single program in each of the inpatient, outpatient, and extended care areas—and for inpatient, that program is Geriatric Consultation, specifically targeting prevention, recognition, and management of inpatient delirium.
Finally, the Deputy Under Secretary for Health for Operations and Management last month approved the formation of a Delirium Field Advisory Committee, charged with advising the GEC office on projects, programs, and activities that hold promise for enhancing awareness of and familiarity about delirium on the part of providers across the continuum of care.	
There is a potential for diagnosis of delirium with some of the tools reviewed. There is some low level evidence of preventive medications and possibly staff education that are useful in preventing delirium. The prevention of delirium could affect performance measures such as length of stay, length of ICU stay, decrease in morbidity, and decrease in NHPPD. This could have a positive impact on patient flow and improved discharge to home settings.	
The annual American Delirium Society conference and EES conferences during the last 3 years will be significantly impacted by these findings. In general, studies in the VA are nearly non-existent, yet VA eligible, VA using patients are sicker than any others in the country (Kazis data). In particular, younger veterans (Vietnam Era) have significant loads of comorbidity (often associated with PTSD as a contributing factor) and really need to be included in the "high risk" category although they don't meet usual age criteria. We may also see a need for OEF/OIF vets to be included for the same reason.	

Delirium: Screening, Prevention, and Diagnosis – A Systematic Review of the Evidence

REVIEWER COMMENT	RESPONSE
Inpatient nurses provide direct care to patients with delirium. The evidence in this report about non-pharmacological interventions to prevent delirium will be especially relevant to nurses in the acute care setting. Once the report is released, the Office of Nursing Field Advisory Committee to discuss how the information from this report on evidence-based nonpharmacological interventions can be disseminated to staff nurses and how we might enlist facilities to trial these evidence-based interventions.	
This report has the potential to impact the standard of care relative to screening of older Veterans for delirium at point of care.	
There is an ongoing quality improvement project in 5 – 7 ICUs measuring CAM ICU and RASS scores	
5. Please provide any recommendations on how this report can be revised to more directly address or assist implementation needs.	
Screening a. In the executive summary, it needs to explicitly state that studies are required in this area to improve detection	**Screening** a. The Future Research section indicates the need for a study of screening.
b. The executive summary and document could use the information contained to highlight the incidence/prevalence of delirium. The goal is to make the statement that this is a common condition	b. We have added incidence/prevalence data to the background section of the executive summary and full report.

c. Targeting – who should the screening target (again using the EBR)
   o Older
   o Cognitively impaired
   o Sensory impairment
	c. The purpose of the evidence review is to present the evidence so that others make informed recommendations.

d. Based on discussion/findings at a recent international meeting, it is fair to de-emphasize the CAM or at least include the requirement for additional mental status testing.	d. Our report is based on published evidence.
e. On Page 14, there is a list of 'indirect links' – prevention needs to be added to this list	e. We have considered this suggestion but believe that prevention is not part of the indirect link. If a preventive strategy has been started, continued assessment of the patient would be considered monitoring of the success of the preventive strategy.
Prevention a. This review is incomplete by only 6-7 papers which were excluded based on a Cochrane review. These papers are described in the text, but not in the analysis and tables – Why not include them in this EBR to produce the most current EBR possible? o It is probably most important around the Marcantonio 2001 trial – which is extensively described	**Prevention** a. We have added the papers from the Cochrane Review and the NICE Guideline that met our study inclusion criteria.
b. The NICE guidelines (published 2 wks ago) are referenced. Did they include the methods (same issue different paper)?	b. We have reviewed this document.
c. While this section focuses on prevention, the results of the rivastigmine in the ICU trial for delirium treatment (stopped due to increased mortality) might be important to cite/mention.	c. We have reviewed the trial mentioned by the reviewer but have not included it in our review because rivastigmine was used for treatment, not for prevention.
d. Why was Kalisvaart's study not included in the meta analysis?)	d. We have added the Kalisvaart study.
e. There are at least two other studies in press on acetylcholinesterase inhibitors and delirium prevention (boustani and marcantonio)	e. As noted above, our inclusion criteria required articles be published in peer review manuscripts.
f. The limited evidence on general vs. regional anesthesia is surprising – consider reviewing Mason SE. J Alz Dis 2010;22;67-79	f. We have reviewed this systematic review and have included 1 study that we had not already identified that met our inclusion criteria.
g. The risks and benefits of the non-pharmacological interventions should be mentioned (low risk interventions)	g. Thank you for this suggestion. We have noted this in the report.

REVIEWER COMMENT	RESPONSE
Diagnosis a. The CAM requires supplemental mental status testing prior to completion. All validation studies of the CAM have completed the MMSE prior to completion. b. This needs to describe / inform about the education and training needed to complete these instruments and diagnose delirium. This is not 'off the shelf' stuff	**Diagnosis** a., b.. These are important points and we have included this information in the findings for KQ3 and the conclusions.
Conclusions a. De-emphasize CAM b. Highlight need for screening studies, limited evidence on pharm interventions, and education / training for diagnosis. Thus there is a strong need for additional studies and additional instruments for this disease	**Conclusions** a., b. Thank you for the suggestions. We have attempted to address them in the Conclusions and Future Research Needs sections.
The report points out the great amount of evidence in the field that is nonetheless non-definitive in its clinical application. The VA population (see above) really does require separate investigation. See Comments below.	We agree that the findings are generally of low-quality and/or insufficient.
Given the evidence presented, it is clear that much more research is needed to identify valid and reliable means of improving detection of delirium. A screening measure that can be universally implemented is needed. The CAM alone does not seem sufficient for this purpose – it requires supplemental mental status testing prior to completion. (Key Question #3)	We again emphasize that there are no data about the effectiveness and harms of screening for delirium in hospitalized medical patients. Therefore, we disagree that a screening measure that can be universally implemented is needed (or at least that such an instrument "should be implemented"). The current evidence does not permit making recommendations on who to screen.
Recommendations for who to screen based on currently available evidence (older, sensory or cognitively impaired) should be highlighted. (Key Question #1)	
More emphasis may also be placed on the non-pharmacological interventions for delirium prevention based in the evidence. These are low-cost, low-risk interventions.(Key Question #2)	We have added a table of risk ratios for the non-pharmacological interventions and more detail about the components of the multi-component interventions.
Limited evidence was reviewed regarding the need for education among providers that fail to recognize delirium across settings where Veterans receive care. (Key Question #1)	We have attempted to address this in the Key Question 1 conclusions.
Flip questions 1 and 3. In the summary, when a reader starts with "no convincing improvement in clinical outcomes, no convincing difference with different drugs, …. Many people won't get to 3. They want validation that their standard of care is fine. There is a way to measure brain dysfunction (which we call delirium like in the 18th century).	The questions are listed in the order originally agreed upon. No further change.
Additional Comments:	
I think this was a very thorough review of the literature and it was disheartening to see that there is little substantiated evidence on screening, identification and prevention of delirium. I did find 2 typos – page 18, first paragraph, states "following up" should state "follow up" Page 37 – typo of control group "if"29-60% and should be control group "of" 29-60%	Thank you for your comments. We have corrected the typos.
Investigations regarding deliriums that may be provoked ONLY by certain medication use (in the absence of other causes) would be very helpful; they may well have different prognoses than the multifactorial ones. This could help greatly because it would offer some "clean" recommendations that could easily be implemented very quickly through the VA.	Thank you for the suggestion. We have included this in the Future Research section.

Screening ... and Diagnosis - A Systematic Review of the Evidence

REVIEWER COMMENT	RESPONSE
This is an important and complex topic for all staff who care for Veterans with delirium, in particular nursing staff who are with these Veterans 24/7 and understand the profound distress this condition causes for both Veterans and their family members. My comments are as follows:	
Introduction-page 4	
Para 1: The 3 reasons that this review was undertaken are not listed in the order that the 3 key questions are discussed throughout this report (same inconsistency appears in the first paragraph of the Executive Summary)	We have corrected to ensure consistency.
Para 2: The authors state that they were "careful to make important distinctions between screening for delirium and diagnosis of delirium." This distinction is somewhat confusing in that the discussion of screening (para 1, page 13) suggests that the purpose of screening is to detect a condition before symptoms occur and the CAM is mentioned as a screen for delirium. Later, however, in the discussion of KQ3, CAM is discussed as a diagnostic tool (Key Question #3). Since the CAM items all address identifiable symptoms, is the CAM a screening test or a diagnostic tool or both? Are there any screening instruments for delirium that detect delirium in the preclinical state? Or are the delirium "screening instruments" really diagnostic instruments (tools)?	CAM could be used as both as a screening instrument in hospitalized patients (individuals without identifiable signs or symptoms of delirium) or as a diagnostic tool (patients with some signs or symptoms that are consistent with but not definitely determined to be delirium (e.g., a patient with confusion). KQ1 and the overarching goal of this report was to assess the effectiveness and harms as a screening tool including in individuals who may be at increased risk due to patient factors (e.g., age, personal history of delirium), index disease type or severity (e.g., stroke, ICU) or co-existing medical conditions/medications that are not directly the reason for admission (e.g. use of narcotics in a patient admitted for COPD). KQ3 assessed the use of CAM as both a diagnostic and screening tool as many of the studies evaluated patients with signs/symptoms potentially compatible with delirium.
Background (page 4)	
In the 3rd sentence, paragraph 4, underlying <u>causes</u> of delirium are listed. The next sentence mentions "<u>risk</u> <u>factors</u>." Are underlying causes of delirium different from risk factors? Is so, what are the risk factors for delirium? Are orthopedic and cardiac surgeries risk factors for delirium or underlying causes of delirium? Most of the pharmacological studies discussed in KQ2 targeted patients who underwent either cardiac or orthopedic surgery yet surgery is not mentioned in para 4 on page 13 either as an underlying cause or risk factor for delirium.	We clarified our use of the term "risk factors". Causality is a strong term that definitely ascribes the outcome to the risk factor. We have clarified regarding surgery.
Key Question 1 (page 13)	
There is no discussion of who (MD, nurse, other staff?) would likely perform screening. In the screening studies/guidelines reviewed, was there mention of who completes the screening? This is an important question given that often the first contact a patient has in the inpatient setting is with a nurse.	This is a policy issue beyond the scope of the review. Screening if found to be effective could be implemented by several lines of health care staff including nurses and physicians and could be done at the admitting floor or in the clinic/emergency room where the admission decision was made. If screening for delirium is effective then future research should be conducted to assess the most effective/efficient methods for implementation.

REVIEWER COMMENT	RESPONSE
Key Question 2 **Pharmacolgocial Studies** Several different pharmacologic studies are discussed (pages 21-24 and 30-31). Most of the pharmacological studies with the exception of Dautezenberg et al (cholinesterase inhibitor) target patients who either underwent orthopedic or cardiac surgery. The report Conclusions on page 45 state, "Low level evidence suggests that pharmacologic strategies using analgesia via fascia iliaca compartmental block, antipsychotic, and lighter anesthesia may be useful in delirium prevention." • Since there are many causes of and many risk factors for delirium, would these pharmacological strategies be useful for "delirium prevention" as stated on page 45 or more specifically would they be useful for delirium prevention in patients undergoing surgical procedures? • The conclusion regarding pharmacological intervention on page 45 seems to imply that these pharmacological interventions would be useful in all patients with delirium when the studies targeted ortho and cardiac surgical patients.	We have clarified regarding surgery.
Non-pharmacological Studies On page 25 the report mentions that 9 multi-component studies consisted of interventions that significantly decrease the incidence of delirium. In the report Conclusions (page 45), multi-component interventions are again mentioned. It might be helpful for those staff interested in implementing multi-component interventions if examples were given of the intervention bundles trialed in some of these studies.	We have added information about the interventions in the multi-component studies.

Overall Organization
 While the discussion of each key question requires a somewhat different approach, there seems to be some inconsistencies in the overall organization of this report.
 1. 1. Each of the key questions has multiple parts.
    a. On page 1, only the subparts of KQ 3 are designated as "a" and "b"
    b. While on page 2, the 4 subparts of KQ 2 are not designated as a-d, on pages 21-35, the subparts are designated as a-d.
    c. The 3 subparts of KQ1 are never designated as a-c.
 2. KQ#1 ends with a "Conclusion"; KQ#2 ends with a "Summary of Finding"; and KQ3 ends abruptly with no conclusions or summary of findings.
	We have corrected these inconsistencies.

Page 6/88 Key Question #1. Consider adding the positives… Lacking direct evidence, ¾ criteria establishing an indirect link between screening and outcomes for delirium were satisfied: 1) patents with delirium have worse outcomes, 2) systematic screening likely improves detection, and 3)harms associated with screening are likely minimal. However, we viewed evidence that treatments for delirium are effective is mixed.	We have modified this section. Without a systematic review of the evidence for each criterion, we are hesitant to say that the criteria were satisfied.
Page 17/88 Paragraph 1. Consider adding after Screening for disease or condition is warranted if the disease is serious …… if treatment or therapeutic decisions would be altered in the presence of the condition.	Thank you – we have modified this statement.
This is an excellent, thorough review that emphasizes the need for research in delirium detection and prevention. I learned a lot by reading it.	Thank you.

APPENDIX D. EVIDENCE TABLES

Appendix D, Table 1: Characteristics of Pharmacologic Prevention Studies

Author, Year, Country, Study Design, Funding Source	Prevention Strategy Used, Controls	Inclusion and Exclusion Criteria, Recruitment Method	Patient Characteristics (expressed in means unless otherwise noted)	Outcomes Evaluated	Study Quality
Randomized trials					
Al-Aama, 2011[37] Canada Study Design: randomized controlled trial (RCT) Funding Source(s): Division of Geriatric Medicine, Department of Medicine, Schulich School of Medicine at The University of Western Ontario	Prevention Strategy Used: melatonin 0.5 mg orally prior to sleep (n=72) Controls: placebo (n=73)	Inclusion Criteria: at least 65 years of age and admitted through the emergency department to Internal Medicine in-patient services Exclusion Criteria: an expected stay or life expectancy of less than 48 hours, were unable to communicate in English or to take oral medications, had an intracranial bleed or seizures, had a markedly non-therapeutic international normalized ratio (INR) less than one or more than four while on warfarin, or had a known allergy to the study compounds Recruitment method: patients were approached directly in the emergency room or in their rooms by one of the three study clinicians within 24 hours of admission (up to 48 h was allowed on weekends)	N=145 Mean age (yrs): 84 Gender, male (%): 43 Race/ethnicity (%): NR Medical unit: Internal Medicine	Incidence of delirium (diagnosed within 6 days post-operatively with the Confusion Assessment Method (CAM)) Delirium severity (Memorial Delirium Assessment Scale) Use of sedatives Use of restraints	Allocation Concealment: adequate (pharmacy controlled) Blinding: double and outcomes assessment Intention to Treat Analysis (ITT): no, 23 patients excluded Withdrawals adequately described: yes
Larsen, 2010[38] US Study Design: RCT Funding Source(s): New England Baptist Hospital Research Department	Prevention Strategy Used: olanzapine 5 mg (oral) (n=243), administered perioperatively Controls: placebo (n=252)	Inclusion Criteria: history of postoperative delirium who were scheduled for elective total knee- or total hip-replacement surgery; ability to speak English; and ability to provide informed consent Exclusion Criteria: a diagnosis of dementia; active alcohol use; a history of alcohol dependence or abuse; allergy to olanzapine; and current use of an antipsychotic medication Recruitment method: NR	N=495 Mean age (yrs): 74 Gender, male (%): 46 Race/ethnicity (%): white 98, non white 2 Medical unit: orthopedic teaching hospital	Incidence of delirium (defined using the Diagnostic and Statistical Manual of Mental Disorders, 3rd edition (DSM-III) Duration of delirium Delirium severity (Severity of delirium according to the highest value of the DRSR-98) Time-to-onset of delirium	Allocation Concealment: adequate (pharmacy controlled) Blinding: double and a independent data and safety monitoring committee evaluated all potentially serious adverse events Intention to Treat Analysis (ITT): no Withdrawals adequately described: yes

Author, Year, Country, Study Design, Funding Source	Prevention Strategy Used, Controls	Inclusion and Exclusion Criteria, Recruitment Method	Patient Characteristics (expressed in means unless otherwise noted)	Outcomes Evaluated	Study Quality
Sieber, 2010[39] US Study Design: RCT Funding Source(s): NA	Prevention Strategy Used: deep sedation with propofol (sedation depth using bispectral index (BIS) of approximately 50) (n=57) Controls: light sedation with propofol (BIS, ≥80) (n=57)	Inclusion Criteria: 65 years or older, undergoing hip fracture repair with spinal anesthesia and propofol sedation Exclusion Criteria: preoperative delirium (determined by CAM); contraindications to spinal anesthesia (e.g., clinically important aortic stenosis, coagulopathy, anticoagulant use, spinal cord disease, refusal of spinal anesthesia), prior hip surgery, severe congestive heart failure (New York Heart Association class IV), severe chronic obstructive pulmonary disease (Global Initiative for Chronic Obstructive Lung Disease guidelines, stage III-IV), or mental or language barriers that would preclude data collection Recruitment method: NR	N=114 Mean age (yrs): 82 Gender, male (%): 27 Race/ethnicity (%): NR Medical unit: multidisciplinary hip fracture service	Incidence of delirium (DSM-III) Delirium duration Time from surgery until discharge Mortality (during hospitalization)	Allocation Concealment: unclear Blinding: double Intention to Treat Analysis (ITT): yes Withdrawals adequately described: yes
Gamberini, 2009[40] Switzerland Study Design: RCT Funding Source(s): Novartis (partial support)	Prevention Strategy Used: rivastigmine (oral) 1.5 mg x 3/day (n=59), starting one day prior to surgery and then post-op for 6 days Controls: placebo (n=61)	Inclusion Criteria: age 65 or older and elective cardiac surgery with cardiopulmonary bypass Exclusion Criteria: urgent or emergency surgery, previous cardiac surgery, cardiac surgery combined with non-cardiac procedures (typically carotid endarterectomy), insufficient knowledge of German or sensory impairment interfering with neuropsychological testing, a preoperative Mini-Mental State Examination (MMSE) <15, psychiatric illness necessitating regular use of antidepressants or antipsychotics, preexisting neurologic deficits, previous or ongoing treatment with cholinesterase inhibitors, and known contraindications for rivastigmine Recruitment method: patients screened for eligibility based on the operation schedule for the following day	N=120, demographic information for 113 patients Mean age (yrs): 74 Gender, male (%): 68 Race/ethnicity (%): NR Medical unit: cardiac surgery	Incidence of delirium (diagnosed within 6 days post-operatively with the CAM) Rescue medication use	Allocation Concealment: adequate, (hospital pharmacy using identical bottles) Blinding: double Intention to Treat Analysis (ITT): no, 7 excluded from analyses Withdrawals adequately described: yes

Author, Year, Country, Study Design, Funding Source	Prevention Strategy Used, Controls	Inclusion and Exclusion Criteria, Recruitment Method	Patient Characteristics (expressed in means unless otherwise noted)	Outcomes Evaluated	Study Quality
Hudetz, 2009[41] US (Veterans) Study Design: RCT Funding Source(s): National Institutes of Health, United States Public Health Service, Medical College of Wisconsin Institutional Grant, departmental funds	Prevention Strategy Used: ketamine 0.5mg/ kg intravenous bolus (n=29) Controls: placebo (n=29) ketamine or placebo administered during anesthetic induction in the presence of fentanyl and etomidate	Inclusion Criteria: at least 55 years of age, provided written informed consent before the initiation of any study-related procedures, scheduled for elective coronary artery bypass graft surgery or valve replacement/repair procedures with cardiopulmonary bypass; patients receiving antidepressants, stimulants, mood stabilizers, anxiolytics, or depressants were eligible Exclusion Criteria: history of cerebrovascular accident within 3 years of randomization, permanent ventricular pacing, previously defined cognitive deficits, patients receiving psychoactive drugs for the treatment of psychosis, hepatic impairment, chronic renal insufficiency, other pre-existing diseases deemed by the investigators to place the patient at an increased risk of perioperative complications Recruitment method: NR	N=58 Mean age (yrs): 64 Gender, male (%): 100 Race/ethnicity (%): white 90 Medical unit: cardiac surgery	Incidence of delirium (Intensive Care Delirium Screening Checklist) Length of stay	Allocation Concealment: unclear ("sealed envelopes") Blinding: double and outcomes assessment Intention to Treat Analysis (ITT): yes Withdrawals adequately described: no withdrawals
Maldonado, 2009[42] US Study Design: RCT Funding Source(s): none stated	Prevention Strategy Used: dexmedetomidine (loading dose: 0.4 µg/kg, followed by a maintenance drip of 0.2 µg/kg/hr–0.7 µg/kg/hr) (n=40) Controls: propofol: 25–50 µg/kg /min (n=38) midazolam: 0.5–2 mg/hr (n=40) All administered postoperatively	Inclusion Criteria: patients undergoing cardiac-valve operations with cardio-pulmonary bypass Exclusion Criteria: preexisting diagnosis of dementia or schizophrenia, the preoperative use of psychotropic medications, active or recent substance abuse or dependence, age less than 18 or older than 90 years, documented stroke within the last 6 months, evidence of advanced heart block, pregnancy, or anticipated intraoperative deep hypothermic circulatory arrest Recruitment method: NR	N=118 Mean age (yrs): 58 Gender, male (%): 64 Race/ethnicity (%): NR Medical unit: cardiac surgery	Incidence of delirium (DSM-IV) Length of stay (hospital and ICU) Rescue medication use (management of delirium) Mortality	Allocation Concealment: unclear Blinding: open-label Intention to Treat Analysis (ITT): no, 28 patients excluded (24%) Withdrawals adequately described: yes

63

Delirium: Screening, Prevention, and Diagnosis – A Systematic Review of the Evidence

Author, Year, Country, Study Design, Funding Source	Prevention Strategy Used, Controls	Inclusion and Exclusion Criteria, Recruitment Method	Patient Characteristics (expressed in means unless otherwise noted)	Outcomes Evaluated	Study Quality
Mouzopolous, 2009[43] Greece Study Design: RCT Funding Source(s): NR	Prevention Strategy Used: fascia iliaca compartment block (FICB) (n=102) - bupivicaine (0.3 mL/kg) 0.25 mg dose of on admission and repeated daily every 24 h until delirium occurrence or hip surgery was performed; 24 hours after hip surgery the same dose of FICB was re-administered and repeated daily every 24 h until delirium occurrence or discharge Controls: placebo (n=105)	Inclusion Criteria: Age 70 years and older admitted for hip fracture Exclusion Criteria: Delirium at admission, metastatic hip cancer, history of bupivicaine allergy, use of cholinesterase inhibitors, severe coagulopathy, Parkinsonism, epilepsy, levodopa treatment, delay of surgery of more than 72 h after admission, and inability to participate in interviews (profound dementia, respiratory isolation, intubation, aphasia, coma or terminal illness) Recruitment method: potentially eligible patients identified by systematically screening new admissions to one orthopedic ward	N=219, demographic information for 207patients Mean age (yrs): 73 Gender, male (%): 26 Race/ethnicity (%): NR Medical unit: orthopedics Risk classification based on 4 predictive risk factors: (1) severity of illness, measured using acute physiology age and chronic health examination; (2) cognitive impairment, measured using the mini-mental state examination score; (3) index of dehydration, measured using the ratio of blood urea nitrogen to creatinine; and (4) visual impair-ment, measured using the standardized Snellen test High risk defined as presence of three or more risk factors	Incidence of delirium (DSM-IV and CAM) Delirium severity (Severity of delirium according to the highest value of the DRSR-98) Delirium duration	Allocation Concealment: adequate, placebo identical in appearance to the active drug and was administered at the same site and in the same way as the FICB Blinding: patients blinded Intention to Treat Analysis (ITT): no, 12 excluded from analyses Withdrawals adequately described: yes

Author, Year, Country, Study Design, Funding Source	Prevention Strategy Used, Controls	Inclusion and Exclusion Criteria, Recruitment Method	Patient Characteristics (expressed in means unless otherwise noted)	Outcomes Evaluated	Study Quality
Prakanrattana, 2007[44] Thailand Study Design: RCT Funding Source(s): Non-industry (Siriraj Grant for Research Development)	Prevention Strategy Used: risperidone 1 mg (sublingual) when regaining consciousness post-op (n=63) Controls: placebo (n=63)	Inclusion Criteria: aged 40 years or older undergoing elective cardiac surgery with cardiopulmonary bypass Exclusion Criteria: patients undergoing emergency surgery, admitted to intensive care unit, tracheal intubation before arriving to operating room, patients experiencing preoperative delirium, history of psychiatric disorders Recruitment method: NR	N=126 Mean age (yrs): 61 Gender, male (%): 59 Race/ethnicity (%): NR Medical unit: cardiac surgery ICU	Incidence of delirium (CAM)	Allocation Concealment: possibly (no identical sublingual placebo but nurses taking care of the patient and assessing delirium left patient bedside to ensure blinding) Blinding: double Intention to Treat Analysis (ITT): yes Withdrawals adequately described: none reported
Sampson, 2007[45] UK Study Design: RCT Funding Source(s): Pfizer Esai, UK	Prevention Strategy Used: donepezil 5mg (n=21), following surgery and every day post-op x 3 days Controls: placebo (n=15)	Inclusion Criteria: patients undergoing elective total hip replacement Exclusion Criteria: patients with mini-mental state examination (MMSE) scores of < 26; patients with sensory impairment who could not undertake neuropsychological testing and those with known hypersensitivity to donepezil or piperidine derivatives or contraindications to the use of donepezil Recruitment method: all patients undergoing elective total hip replacement and attending the pre-admission assessment clinic, who were able to give informed consent, were invited to participate	N=50; demographic information for 33 patients Mean age (yrs): 68 Gender, male (%): 52 Race/ethnicity (%): NR Medical unit: orthopedics	Incidence of delirium (as indicated by the Delirium Symptom Interview) Length of hospital stay	Allocation Concealment: adequate, by the hospital pharmacy Blinding: double, and data were analyzed blind to randomization code Intention to Treat Analysis (ITT): no; 14 withdrawn after randomization; 3 excluded after treatment allocation Withdrawals adequately described: yes

Author, Year, Country, Study Design, Funding Source	Prevention Strategy Used, Controls	Inclusion and Exclusion Criteria, Recruitment Method	Patient Characteristics (expressed in means unless otherwise noted)	Outcomes Evaluated	Study Quality
Kalisvaart, 2005[46] The Netherlands Study Design: RCT Funding Source(s): NR	Prevention Strategy Used: haloperidol 1.5 mg/d (n=212), started preoperatively and continued for up to 3 days postoperatively Controls: placebo (n=218)	Inclusion Criteria: aged 70 and older admitted for acute/ elective hip surgery and were at intermediate or high risk for postoperative delirium Exclusion Criteria: delirium at admission, no risk factors for postoperative delirium present at baseline, history of haloperidol allergy, use of cholinesterase inhibitors, parkinsonism, epilepsy, levodopa treatment, inability to participate in interviews, delay of surgery > 72 hours after admission, or a prolonged QTc interval of 460 ms or higher for men and 470 ms or higher for women on their electro-cardiogram Recruitment method: a research team of geriatricians and nurses in a single 915- bed teaching hospital identified potentially eligible patients by systematically screening new admissions to two surgical and three orthopedic wards	N=430 Mean age (yrs): 79 Gender, male (%): 20 Race/ethnicity (%): NR Medical unit: Surgical and orthopedic wards Risk classification based on presence of four predictive risk factors: (1) Visual impairment (binocular near vision worse than 20/70 after correction); (2) severity of illness, measured using the Acute Physiology Age and Chronic Health Examination (score of 16 or higher indicating increased severity); (3) cognitive impairment (MMSE score ≤ 24 on a scale of 0–30); and (4) index of dehydration (ratio of blood urea nitrogen to creatinine of ≥18) Intermediate risk -presence of 1or 2 risk factors High risk - presence of ≥ 3 risk factors	Incidence of post-operative delirium (DSM IV and Confusion Assessment Method criteria) Delirium duration Delirium severity (measured using the Delirium Rating Scale (DRS), revised version-98, range 0 (no severity) to 45 (high severity)). Length of stay	Allocation Concealment: adequate (hospital pharmacist had prepackaged) Blinding: double and members of the research team not involved in the clinical care of the patients performed all baseline and outcome assessments Intention to Treat Analysis (ITT): yes Withdrawals adequately described: yes

Author, Year, Country, Study Design, Funding Source	Prevention Strategy Used, Controls	Inclusion and Exclusion Criteria, Recruitment Method	Patient Characteristics (expressed in means unless otherwise noted)	Outcomes Evaluated	Study Quality
Liptzin, 2005[47] US Study Design: RCT Funding Source(s): Pfizer Corporation	Prevention Strategy Used: donepezil 14 days before and after surgery (n=39) Controls: placebo (n=41)	Inclusion Criteria: scheduled for elective total knee or hip arthroplasty and aged 50 or greater; able to give informed consent Exclusion Criteria: evidence of gastroesophageal reflux disease or sick-sinus syndrome; currently taking donepezil or previously intolerant of it; did not speak English; already in another trial Recruitment method: recruited from pts scheduled for elective total hip or knee arthroplasty	N=90 (Baseline info for 80; 58 completed trial) Mean age (yrs): 67 Gender, male (%): 43 Race/ethnicity (%): white 97.5, other 2.5 Medical unit: orthopedic surgery	Incidence of delirium (DSM-IV) Mean duration of post-op delirium Number with post-op subsyndromal delirium Mean duration of subsyndromal delirium Mean length of stay	Allocation Concealment: adequate (by pharmacist) Blinding: double Intention to Treat Analysis (ITT): no, 10 not operated on were excluded Withdrawals adequately described: yes
Papaioannou, 2005[48] Greece Study Design: RCT Funding Source(s): European Commission's BIOMED2 program BMH4-98-3335 and Greek Ministry of Health.	Prevention Strategy Used: regional anesthesia (epidural or spinal) (n=25) Controls: general anesthesia (n=25)	Inclusion Criteria: aged at least 60 years, scheduled for elective surgery that could be performed under regional or general anesthesia and who had agreed to be randomly allocated to receive either type of anesthesia Exclusion Criteria: illiteracy, severe auditory or visual disturbances, central nervous system disorders, alcoholism or drug dependence, treatment with tranquilizers or antidepressants, Parkinson's disease and a preoperative MMSE score ≤ 23 points, indicative of dementia Recruitment method: NR	N=50 (Baseline info for 47) Median age (yrs): 68 Gender, male (%): 64 Race/ethnicity (%): NR Medical unit: surgery (orthopedic and vascular)	Incidence of delirium (DSM-III)	Allocation Concealment: unclear Blinding: none stated Intention to Treat Analysis (ITT): no, 3 patients were excluded Withdrawals adequately described: yes
Aizawa, 2002[49] Japan Study Design: RCT Funding Source(s): none stated	Prevention Strategy Used: delirium free protocol, post surgery; diazepam 0.1 mg/kg IM at 20;00; flunitrazepam 0.04 mg/kg and pethidine 1 mg/kg continuous IV infusions for 8 hours x 3 nights (n=20) Controls: usual care (n=20)	Inclusion Criteria: patients aged over 70 but less than 86 years of age who underwent resection of gastric or colorectal cancer through an open laparotomy under general anesthesia Exclusion Criteria: liver cirrhosis or liver dysfunction, renal dysfunction, respiratory disturbance, other poor risk factors, mental disorders, visual impairment, or patients who required extensive resection of other organs or emergency surgery Recruitment method: NR	N=42 (Baseline info for 40; 2 excluded due to incomplete administration of agents) Mean age (yrs): 76 Gender, male (%): 65 Race/ethnicity (%): NR Medical unit: surgery	Incidence of delirium (DSM-IV) Mean length of stay	Allocation Concealment: unclear Blinding: outcomes assessor Intention to Treat Analysis (ITT): no, 2 were excluded Withdrawals adequately described: yes

Delirium: Screening, Prevention, and Diagnosis – A Systematic Review of the Evidence

Author, Year, Country, Study Design, Funding Source	Prevention Strategy Used, Controls	Inclusion and Exclusion Criteria, Recruitment Method	Patient Characteristics (expressed in means unless otherwise noted)	Outcomes Evaluated	Study Quality
Williams-Russo, 1992[13] US Study Design: RCT Funding Source(s): National Institute of Aging	Prevention Strategy Used: continuous epidural bupivicaine and fentanyl infusions (n=26). Initiated post-op at first complaint of pain Controls: continuous intravenous fentanyl infusions (n=25). Initiated post-op at first complaint of pain	Inclusion Criteria: scheduled for a bilateral knee replacement, speak English as a primary language, and have no serious hearing or vision impairment which would preclude cognitive testing Exclusion Criteria: none stated Recruitment method: bilateral knee surgery patients were approached	N=51 Mean age (yrs): 68 Gender, male (%): 45 Race/ethnicity (%): NR Medical unit: Urban referral hospital specializing in elective orthopedic surgery	Incidence of delirium (DSM-III)	Allocation Concealment: unclear Blinding: physicians and nurses administering care not aware of purpose of study; study personnel not involved in patient care/treatment decisions Intention to Treat Analysis (ITT): no Withdrawals adequately described: yes
Kaneko, 1999[50] Japan Study Design: RCT Funding Source(s): Not reported	Prevention Strategy Used: intravenous haloperidol (5 mg in 1.0mL daily) from 1st to 5th post-operative day (n=38) Controls: equal volume of normal saline injection (0.9%) (n=40)	Inclusion Criteria: patients scheduled for elective gastrointestinal surgery, admitted to High and Intensive Care Unit before scheduled surgery Exclusion Criteria: none stated Recruitment method: Iinterviewed after admission	N=80 (2 patients excluded, unclear if excluded before or after randomization) Mean age (yrs): 72.8 Gender, male (%): 63 Race/ethnicity (%): NR Medical unit: high and Intensive Care Unit for gastrointestinal surgery	Incidence of delirium (DSM-III-R)	Allocation Concealment: unclear Blinding: none reported Intention to Treat Analysis (ITT): unclear Withdrawals adequately described: no – unclear when 2 patients were excluded

Author, Year, Country, Study Design, Funding Source	Prevention Strategy Used, Controls	Inclusion and Exclusion Criteria, Recruitment Method	Patient Characteristics (expressed in means unless otherwise noted)	Outcomes Evaluated	Study Quality
Berggren, 1987[51] Sweden Study Design: RCT Funding Source(s): Swedish Medical Research Council, No. 12x-5664, King Gustav V's 80th Birthday Foundation, and the Umei University Research Foundation	Prevention Strategy Used: epidural anesthesia (n=28) Controls: halothane anesthesia (n=29)	Inclusion Criteria: patients admitted to the orthopedic wards for femoral neck fractures and were fully lucid Exclusion Criteria: none stated Recruitment method: NR	N=57 Mean age (yrs): 78 Gender, male (%): 19 Race/ethnicity (%): NR Medical unit: orthopedic wards	Incidence of delirium (DSM-III) Mean length of stay Mortality	Allocation Concealment: unclear Blinding: outcomes assessor Intention to Treat Analysis (ITT): yes Withdrawals adequately described: yes

Non-randomized trials

Author, Year, Country, Study Design, Funding Source	Prevention Strategy Used, Controls	Inclusion and Exclusion Criteria, Recruitment Method	Patient Characteristics (expressed in means unless otherwise noted)	Outcomes Evaluated	Study Quality
Katznelson, 2009[52] Canada Study Design: prospective observational study Funding Source(s): University of Toronto	Prevention Strategy Used: statins (n=676) Controls: no statins (383)	Inclusion Criteria: patients undergoing cardiac surgery Exclusion Criteria: patients undergoing congenital or redo surgery, or requiring circulatory arrest, were excluded Recruitment method: NA	N=1059 Mean age (yrs): NA Gender, male (%): 71 Race/ethnicity (%): NR Medical unit: cardiovascular ICU	Incidence of delirium (diagnosed with CAM), presented as an odds ratio and also stratified by age groups (age <60 years and ≥ 60 years)	Allocation Concealment: Not applicable (NA) Blinding: single blinded (nursing staff) Intention to Treat Analysis (ITT): NA Withdrawals adequately described: NA

Delirium: Screening, Prevention, and Diagnosis – A Systematic Review of the Evidence

Author, Year, Country, Study Design, Funding Source	Prevention Strategy Used, Controls	Inclusion and Exclusion Criteria, Recruitment Method	Patient Characteristics (expressed in means unless otherwise noted)	Outcomes Evaluated	Study Quality
Del Rosario, 2008[53] Spain Study Design: retrospective comparison Funding Source(s): NR	Prevention Strategy Used: patient-controlled femoral nerve analgesia (n=49) Controls: intravenous analgesia (n=50)	Inclusion Criteria: ≥ 50 years old; underwent hip fracture surgery with intradural anesthesia Exclusion Criteria: received general- anesthesia or epidural analgesia, presented failure of femoral analgesia, or had localized infection or coagulopathy Recruitment method: NA, chart review	N=99 Mean age (yrs): 81 Gender, male (%): Intervention: 20, Control: 38, p=0.08 Race/ethnicity (%): NR Medical unit: orthopedics	Incidence of delirium (documentation of altered mental status (confusion, disorientation, changes of level of consciousness, changes in the sleep-wake cycle)) Delirium severity (classified into two degrees of severity, low or severe, according to the need of prescription of any antipsychotic drug) Rescue medication use	Allocation Concealment: NA Blinding: NA Intention to Treat Analysis (ITT): NA Withdrawals adequately described: NA
Dautzenberg, 2004[12] The Netherlands Study Design: Retrospective cohort study Funding Source(s): NR	Prevention Strategy Used: rivastigmine chronic users (n=11) Controls: non-rivastigmine users (n=29)	Inclusion Criteria: patients who were treated by the geriatric consultation team and had the appearance of a delirium or were considered to be at high-risk of develop delirium by their treating physician Exclusion Criteria: NR Recruitment method: group of 366 hospitalized patients, treated by the geriatric consultation team from January 2002 to June 2003, chronic rivastigmine users compared with randomly selected subgroup of all patients not treated with rivastigmine.	N=40 Mean age (yrs): 79 Gender, male (%): 40 Race/ethnicity (%): NR Medical unit: Non-geriatric wards	Diagnosed delirium during the time of hospitalization of the patient (based on DSM-IV criteria, and recorded in the medical record) Length of hospital stay Mortality	Allocation Concealment: NA Blinding: NA Intention to Treat Analysis (ITT): NA Withdrawals adequately described: NA
Savage, 1978[54] US Study Design: non-random comparison Funding Source(s): NR	Prevention Strategy Used: physostigmine (n=45) Controls: No physostigmine (n=68)	Inclusion Criteria: randomly selected pts who underwent elective surgery and were either Status I or II (American Society of Anesthesiologists) Exclusion Criteria: bradycardia, bronchial asthma, obstructive pulmonary disease, pregnancy, Parkinson's Recruitment method: NA	N=113 Mean age (yrs): NR Gender, male (%): NR Race/ethnicity (%): NR Medical unit: surgical	Subjects were evaluated, post-surgery, on the following scale: 1) restless, thrashing, a score of 1; 2) mumbling, incoherent, a score of 2; 3) reacting, quiet, but nonverbal, a score of 3; 4) and appropriate verbal responses, a score of 4	Allocation Concealment: NA Blinding: nurses who graded delirium, were blinded to intervention Intention to Treat Analysis (ITT): NA Withdrawals adequately described: NA

Appendix D, Table 2. Primary Prevention Outcomes of Pharmacologic Studies

Author, Year/ Drug class	Delirium Incidence/ Prevalence n/N (%)		Delirium Severity (SD unless noted)		Delirium Duration, days (SD unless noted)		Length of Stay, days (SD unless noted)		Use of Rescue Medications n/N (%)	
	Intervention	Control	Intervention	Control	Intervention	Control	Intervention	Control	Intervention	Control
Randomized studies										
Al-Aama 2011[37] Melatonin	7/61 (11.5) p=0.01	19/61 (31.1)	MDAS delirium only 10.5 (5.3) p=0.77	delirium only 11.4 (3.0)			18.5 (26.4) p=0.36	14.5 (21.6)	PRN sedatives 33/61 (54.1) p=0.46	PRN sedatives
Larsen 2010[38] Antipsychotic	28/196 (14.3) p<0.0001	82/204 (40.2)	DRSR-98 16.4 (3.7) p=0.02	DRSR-98 14.5 (2.7)	2.2 (1.3) p=0.02	1.6 (0.7)			A trend toward use of fewer narcotics in the intervention arm but difference not significant	
Sieber 2010[39] Anesthesia	Light sed. 11/57 (19) p=0.02	Deep sed. 23/57 (40)	MMSE score 2 days post-op 23.1 (5.5) p=0.08 Change from baseline -2.1 (3.4) p=0.06	MMSE score 2 days post-op 20.0 (9.3) Change from baseline -4.4 (6.1)	Light sed. All 0.5 (1.5) p=0.01 delirium only 2.8 (2.3) p=0.77	Deep sed. All 1.4 (4.0) p=0.01 delirium only 3.4 (5.7)	Light sed. mean 4.7 (3.1) p=0.69	Deep sed. Mean 4.5 (2.3)		
Gamberini 2009[40] Cholinesterase inhibitor	18/56* (32.1) **p=0.79	17/57* (29.8)			Median 2.5 (range 1-5) p=0.30	Median 3 (range 1-5)	Median 13 (range 7-39) p=0.3	Median 13 (range 7-39)	Haloperidol 17/56 (30.4) p=0.90 Lorazepam 35/56 (62.5) p=0.70	Haloperidol 18/57 (30.4) Lorazepam 38/57 (66.7)
Hudetz 2009[41] Anesthesia	1/29 (3.4) p=0.01	9/29 (31.0)					8 (4.0) p=0.36	7 (3.0)		
Maldonado 2009[42] Postoperative sedation	Dexmedet. 4/40 (10.0) p<0.001 both controls *Per protocol* Dexmedet. 1/30 (3.3) p<0.001 both controls	Propofol 16/36 (44.4) Midazolam 17/40 (42.5) *Per protocol* Propofol 15/30 (50.0) Midazolam 15/30 (50.0)			Dexmedet. 2.0 (0.0) p=0.93 vs. propofol, 0.63 vs. midazolam	Propofol 3.0 (3.1) Midazolam 5.4 (6.6)	Dexmedet. 7.1 (1.9) p=0.42 vs. propofol, 0.12 vs. midazolam	Propofol 8.2 (3.8) Midazolam 8.9 (4.7)	Haloperidol Dexmedet. 0/30 p=0.07 vs. propofol, 0.15 vs. midazolam Lorazepam Dexmedet. 1/30 (3.3) p=0.06 vs. propofol, 0.11 vs. midazolam	Haloperidol Propofol 3/30 (10.0) Midazolam 2/30 (6.7) Lorazepam Propofol 7/30 (23.3) Midazolam 6/30 (20.0)

Delirium: Screening, Prevention, and Diagnosis – A Systematic Review of the Evidence

Author, Year / Drug class	Delirium Incidence/ Prevalence n/N (%)		Delirium Severity (SD unless noted)		Delirium Duration, days (SD unless noted)		Length of Stay, days (SD unless noted)		Use of Rescue Medications n/N (%)	
	Intervention	Control	Intervention	Control	Intervention	Control	Intervention	Control	Intervention	Control
Mouzopolous 2009[43] *Analgesia*	All* 11/102 (10.8) p=0.017 High risk group 9/17 (52.9) p=0.73	All* 25/105 (23.8) High risk group 10/16 (62.5)	DRSR-98 Highest value 14.3 (3.6) p<0.001	DRSR-98 Highest value 18.6 (3.4)	5.2 (4.3) p<0.001	11 (7.2)				
Prakanrattana 2007[44] *Antipsychotic*	7/63 (11.1) p=0.01	20/63 (31.7)								
Sampson 2007[45] *Cholinesterase inhibitor*	2/19 (10.5) p=0.08	5/14 (35.7)					9.9 (0.7) p=0.09	12.1 (1.1)		
Kalisvaart, 2005[46] *Antipsychotic*	32/212 (15.1) p=0.69	36/218 (16.5)	Based on DRS, range 0-45 14.4 (3.4) p<0.001	Based on DRS, range 0-45 18.4 (4.3)	5.4 (4.9) p<0.001	11.8 (7.5)	All 13.8 (7.7) p=0.84 Delirious pts. only 17.1 (11.1) p<0.001	All 13.6 (7.8) Delirious pts. only 22.6 (16.7)		
Liptzin 2005[47] *Cholinesterase inhibitor*	DSM-IV 8/39 (20.5) p=0.69 Subsyndromal (Sub) 28/39 (71.8) p=0.57	DSM-IV 7/41 (17.1) Sub. 27/41 (65.8)			DSM-IV 1.0 (SE 0.0) p=0.12 Sub. 1.71 (SE 0.19)	DSM-IV 1.3 (SE 0.19) Sub. 2.04 (SE 0.23)	4.4 (SE 0.13)	4.2 (SE 0.08)		
Papaioannou 2005[48] *Anesthesia*	Regional 3/19†† (15.8) p=0.63	General 6/28†† (21.4)								
Aizawa 2002[49] *Delirium free protocol (DFP) (Benzodiaze-pines)*	DFP 1/20 (5.0) p=0.06 Accidents cause by delirium‡ 1/20 (5.0) p=0.10	Control 7/20 (35.0) Accidents cause by delirium‡ 5/20 (25.0)					DFP 25.6 (9.4) p=0.74	Control 29.9 (16.2)		

Author, Year / Drug class	Delirium Incidence/Prevalence n/N (%)		Delirium Severity (SD unless noted)		Delirium Duration, days (SD unless noted)		Length of Stay, days (SD unless noted)		Use of Rescue Medications n/N (%)	
	Intervention	Control	Intervention	Control	Intervention	Control	Intervention	Control	Intervention	Control
Williams-Russo 1992[13] *Analgesia*	Bupivivicaine +Fentanyl 10/26 (38.4) p=0.69	Fentanyl 11/25 (44.0)								
Kaneko, 1999[50] *Antipsychotic*	4/38 (10.5) p<0.05	13/40 (32.5)								
Berggren 1987[51] *Anesthesia*	Epidural 14/28 (50.0) p=0.36	Halothane 11/29 (37.9)								
Non-randomized studies										
Katznelson, 2009[52] *Antilipid therapy*	All 73/676 (10.8) p=0.33 Age < 60 9/188 (4.8) Age 60+ 64/488(13.1)	All 49/383 (12.8) Age < 60 12/197(6.1) Age 60+ 37/186(19.9)								
Del Rosario 2008[53] *Analgesia*	4/49 (8.2) p<0.001 Severe 0/49	21/50 (42.0) Severe 11/50 (22)					7.7 (3.0) p=0.16	8.6 (3.5)	Opioids 0/49 p<0.001	Opioids 14/50 (28)
Dautzenberg 2004[12] *Cholinesterase inhibitor*	5/11 (45.5) p=0.01	26/29 (88.9)					40.6 (95%CI -20-101.2); p=0.73	28.4 (95%CI (-16.8-73.6)		
Savage 1978[54] *Cholinesterase inhibitor*	Score of 1 or 2† 4/45 (8.9); p<0.01 Score of 1, 2 or 3† 13/45 (28.9); p<0.001	Score of 1 or 2† 29/68 (42.6) Score of 1, 2 or 3† 47/68 (69.1)								

*Number analyzed or completed trial

** All p-values are versus control. If not provided, they were calculated by the reviewers.

† 1 = a restless, thrashing patient, who is a danger to himself and required physical restraint; 2 = mumbling, groaning, incoherent, unresponsive patient; 3 = a reacting, quiet, non-verbal patient; 4 = an awake patent who appropriate verbal responses. / responded to all verbal commands; 4 = an awake patent who appropriate verbal responses.

†† Data were analyzed per protocol. 25 patients each were randomized to the regional and general anesthesia arms, respectively. 4 patients receiving regional anesthesia failed and crossed over to general and 3 patients (2 regional, 1 general) refused to go with study and were then excluded. Final n=47 (19 regional and 28 general).

‡ 5 patients pulled out nasal-gastric tube, one pulled out central vein line, and all showed "strange behavior" like peeling off dressing gauze or fumbling with tubes.

Appendix D, Table 3: Characteristics of Non-Pharmacologic or Mixed Treatments Prevention Studies

Author, Year, Country, Study Design, Funding Source	Prevention Strategy Used, Controls	Inclusion and Exclusion Criteria, Recruitment Method	Patient Characteristics (expressed in means unless otherwise noted)	Outcomes Evaluated	Study Quality
Randomized Trials					
Lundstrom, 2007[55] Sweden Study Design: RCT Funding Source(s): non-industry (Vardal Fdn, Joint Committee of the Northern Health Region of Sweden, JC Kempe Memorial Fdn, Fdn of the Medical Faculty, Univ of Umea, County Council of Vasterbotten, Swedish Research Council)	Prevention Strategy Used: post operative multi-factorial intervention program (n=102); intervention consisted of staff education focusing on the assessment, prevention and treatment of delirium and associated complications Controls: postoperative care in the Orthopedic Department according to the usual postoperative care routines (n=97)	Inclusion Criteria: aged 70 years or older, consecutively admitted to the Orthopedic Department at the University Hospital in Umea, Sweden, between May 2000 and December 2002 with femoral neck fracture Exclusion Criteria: severe rheumatoid arthritis, severe hip osteoarthritis, severe renal failure, pathological fracture, bedridden status prior to fracture Recruitment Method: in emergency room, patients were asked both in writing and orally if they were willing to participate in the study; in the case of patients with cognitive impairment, next-of-kin were also asked	N=199 Mean age (yrs): 82 Gender, male (%): 26 Race/ethnicity (%): NR Medical unit: specialized geriatric ward or conventional orthopedic ward	Delirium prevalence (defined as DSM IV) Delirium duration Length of stay Mortality	Allocation Concealment: yes (sealed and opaque envelopes) Blinding: outcomes assessor Intention to Treat Analysis (ITT): yes Withdrawals adequately described: yes
Taguchi, 2007[56] Japan Study Design: RCT Funding Source(s): NR	Prevention Strategy Used: bright light therapy (n=8) Controls: natural lighting environment (n=7)	Inclusion Criteria: middle-aged or aged patients who had no mental or ophthalmologic disorders and were capable of communication in Japanese Exclusion Criteria: NR Recruitment Method: Patients undergoing surgery for esophageal cancer were recruited	N=15 Mean age (yrs): 58 Gender, male (%): 100 Race/ethnicity (%): NR Medical unit: ICU	Delirium incidence (defined using Japanese version (2001) of the NEECHAM Confusion Scale)	Allocation Concealment: unclear Blinding: NR Intention to Treat Analysis (ITT): no, 4 excluded from analyses Withdrawals adequately described: yes (reintubated patients and patients with complications excluded)

Author, Year, Country, Study Design, Funding Source	Prevention Strategy Used, Controls	Inclusion and Exclusion Criteria, Recruitment Method	Patient Characteristics (expressed in means unless otherwise noted)	Outcomes Evaluated	Study Quality
McCaffrey, 2006[57] United States Study Design: RCT Funding Source(s): NR	Prevention Strategy Used: usual post-operative care plus music (patient's choice from CDs provided) played at least 1 hour, 4 times/day (n=62) Controls: usual post-operative care (no music protocol) (n=62)	Inclusion Criteria: elders undergoing elective hip or knee surgery; over 65 years of age; alert and oriented to provide consent to surgery and to complete preoperative paperwork independently; able to hear music Exclusion Criteria: NA Recruitment Method: recruited during pre-op interview	N=126 (124 completed the study) Mean age (yrs): 77 Gender, male (%): 36 Race/ethnicity (%): NR Medical unit: large tertiary care center (orthopedic)	Delirium incidence (based on review of nurses' notes after patient was discharged)	Allocation Concealment: unclear Blinding: none Intention to Treat Analysis (ITT): no Withdrawals adequately described: yes
Lundstrom, 2005[58] Sweden Study Design: RCT Funding Source(s): Non-industry (Joint Committee of the Northern Health Region of Sweden and others)	Prevention Strategy Used: intervention ward (n=200); multi-component including education in geriatric medicine focusing on assessment, prevention, and treatment of delirium, education concerning caregiver-patient interaction focusing on patients with dementia and delirium, reorganization from a task-allocation care system to a patient-allocation system with individualized care, monthly guidance for nursing staff Controls: control ward care (usual hospital care) (n=200)	Inclusion Criteria: aged 70 and older Exclusion Criteria: patient refusal Recruitment Method: patients mainly (93.8%) admitted from the emergency room in the same proportion to each ward	N=400 Mean age (yrs): 80.1 Gender, male (%): 44 Race/ethnicity (%): NR Medical unit: general internal medicine	Delirium incidence, (defined by DSM-IV) Delirium duration	Allocation Concealment: unclear Blinding: outcomes assessor Intention to Treat Analysis (ITT): yes Withdrawals adequately described: all included
Marcantonio, 2001[59] United States Study Design: RCT Funding Source(s): Older Americans Independence Center; Charles Farnsworth Trust	Prevention Strategy Used: proactive geriatrics consultation, preoperatively or within 24 hours of surgery (n=62) Controls: Usual care (n=64)	Inclusion Criteria: patients 65 years or older admitted for primary surgical repair of hip fracture Exclusion Criteria: presence of metastatic cancer or other comorbid illness likely to reduce life expectancy to less than 6 months, or inability to give informed consent within 24 hours of surgery or 48 hours from admission Recruitment Method: patients approached by investigators after admitted	N=126 Mean age (yrs): 79 Gender, male (%): 21 Race/ethnicity (%): white 90 Medical unit: orthopedic surgery	Delirium incidence (CAM) Severe delirium incidence (CAM-defined delirium with MDAS score ≥18) Delirium duration Length of stay	Allocation Concealment: unclear ("sealed envelopes") Blinding: outcomes assessor for delirium incidence Intention to Treat Analysis (ITT): yes Withdrawals adequately described: all included

Delirium: Screening, Prevention, and Diagnosis – A Systematic Review of the Evidence

Author, Year, Country, Study Design, Funding Source	Prevention Strategy Used, Controls	Inclusion and Exclusion Criteria, Recruitment Method	Patient Characteristics (expressed in means unless otherwise noted)	Outcomes Evaluated	Study Quality
Non-randomized studies					
Ushida, 2009[60] Japan Study Design: Prospective cohort with retrospective control Funding Source(s): None	Prevention Strategy Used: postoperative care under modified protocols were prospectively examined (n=41) Controls: cervical myelopathy patients were retrospectively examined about the incidence of post-operative delirium (n=81)	Inclusion Criteria: patients who met indication criteria for cervical decompression surgery Exclusion Criteria: dementia, other psychological disorders Recruitment Method: NA	N=122 Mean age (yrs): Intervention: 68 Control: 70 Gender, male (%): NR Race/ethnicity (%): NR Medical unit: neurology (spinal surgery)	Delirium incidence (based on DSM-IV criteria)	Allocation Concealment: NA Blinding: NA Intention to Treat Analysis (ITT): NA Withdrawals adequately described: NA
Vidan, 2009[61] Spain Study Design: Non-randomized controlled clinical trial Funding Source(s): Non-industry (Spanish Geriatrics Society)	Prevention Strategy Used: quality improvement program with two major components: an educational program aimed at changing the approach of geriatric ward staff to patient care and a set of specific targeted actions in 7 risk factor domains (orientation, sensorial perception, sleep preservation, mobilization, hydration, nutrition, drug list review) (n=172) Controls: standard care provided by internists, nurses, and additional staff (nutritionists, rehabilitation team, social workers), when needed (n=372)	Inclusion Criteria: aged 70 and older, with any of the risk criteria for delirium (cognitive impairment, visual impairment, acute disease severity, dehydration) Exclusion Criteria: presence of severe dementia that impaired communication, aphasia of any origin, coma, agonic status, or expected hospital stay less than 48 hours Recruitment Method: patients who did not have delirium at the time of admission and had ≥ 1 of the four risk factors of delirium (cognitive impairment, visual impairment, acute disease severity, and dehydration) were included	N=542 Mean age (yrs): Intervention: 86 Control: 82 p<0.001 Gender, male (%): Intervention: 38 Control: 47 p=0.04 Race/ethnicity (%): NR Medical unit: Internal medicine or geriatrics *Note: there were significant differences (p<0.05)in several of the baseline characteristics*	Delirium incidence (defined according to the criteria of the CAM) Delirium severity (measured using an additive score for the four delirium symptoms included in the CAM; evaluator rated each delirium symptom, except fluctuation, as absent (0 points), mild (1 point), or severe (2 points); fluctuation was rated as absent (0 points) or present (1 point); sum of these points ranged from 0 to 7 with higher scores indicating greater severity) Delirium duration Mortality	Allocation Concealment: NA Blinding: A trained research assistant, who was not involved in the intervention, conducted all interviews. Intention to Treat Analysis (ITT): yes Withdrawals adequately described: NA

Author, Year, Country, Study Design, Funding Source	Prevention Strategy Used, Controls	Inclusion and Exclusion Criteria, Recruitment Method	Patient Characteristics (expressed in means unless otherwise noted)	Outcomes Evaluated	Study Quality
Kratz, 2008[62] United States Study Design: quasi-experimental Funding Source(s): none stated	Prevention Strategy Used: acute confusion (AC) protocol, an evidence-based project which focused on 3 protocols (1) patient orientation (2) non-pharmacologic sleep; and (3) early mobilization; implemented by an interdisciplinary team (pharmacists, occupational therapists, physical therapists, nurses, and nurses' aides) Pilot study: two units each chose an intervention to implement for 1 month Following pilot study, implementation of all 3 protocols was initiated Controls: pilot study: one unit continued usual care of the elderly	Inclusion Criteria: 70 years or older, admitted for more than 23 hours, and without a communication barrier or having an alcohol withdrawal experience Exclusion Criteria: none stated Recruitment Method: NA	N=137 (pilot study) Mean age (yrs): NR, all >70 years of age Gender, male (%): NR Race/ethnicity (%): NR Medical unit: medical/surgical	Delirium (AC) incidence in the pilot study Rate of falls Use of restraints Usage of anti-anxiety medications (known to cause acute confusion)	Allocation Concealment: NA Blinding: NA Intention to Treat Analysis (ITT): NA Withdrawals adequately described: NA
Robinson, 2008[63] Vollmer, 2007[64] United States Study Design: pre- and post-intervention study; data collected using retrospective record review Funding Source(s): none stated	Prevention Strategy Used: delirium protocol - interventions from the HELP program and strategies suggested by Foreman et al. (2003)* - implemented in a post-intervention group; interventions implemented by nursing assistants and included specific approaches for patients with dementia, hearing impairment, vision impairment, and mobility impairment (n=80) Controls: matched convenience sample of patients over the age of 65 with any combination of the risk factors of the post-intervention group who were admitted prior to the implementation of the delirium prevention protocol (n=80) *Foreman MD, Mion LC, Trygstad LJ, Fletcher K. (2003). Delirium: Strategies for assessing and treating. In M. Mezey, et al. (Eds.). Geriatric nursing protocols for best practice (2nd ed., pp. 63–75). New York: Springer.	Inclusion Criteria: over the age of 65 with any combination of the risk factors of dementia, vision impairment, hearing impairment, and mobility impairment Exclusion Criteria: NR Recruitment Method: on admission, patients over 65 were assessed for risk factors of dementia, vision impairment, hearing impairment, and mobility impairment by the registered nurse admitting the patient	N=160 Mean age (yrs): Pre-intervention (control) group: 79.2 Post-intervention group: 78.8 Gender, male (%):46% Race/ethnicity (%): NR Medical unit: renal	Delirium incidence (defined according to the criteria of the CAM)	Allocation Concealment: NA Blinding: NA Intention to Treat Analysis (ITT): NA Withdrawals adequately described: NA

Delirium: Screening, Prevention, and Diagnosis – A Systematic Review of the Evidence

Author, Year, Country, Study Design, Funding Source	Prevention Strategy Used, Controls	Inclusion and Exclusion Criteria, Recruitment Method	Patient Characteristics (expressed in means unless otherwise noted)	Outcomes Evaluated	Study Quality
Caplan, 2007[65] Australia Study Design: controlled before-and-after study Funding Source(s): Non-industry (Commonwealth Department of Health and Aging)	Prevention Strategy Used: volunteer-mediated intervention of daily orientation, therapeutic activities, feeding and hydration assistance, vision and hearing protocols based on the Hospital Elder Life Program (HELP) developed at Yale University School of Medicine; training materials purchased through the HELP mentorship program and adapted to POWH so that the whole intervention could be delivered by volunteers; volunteer coordinator employed to select, train and oversee volunteers delivering a set of interventions to elderly patients (n=16) Controls: usual care (n=21)	Inclusion Criteria: at least one of the following risk factors for developing delirium: mini-mental state examination < 24, sleep deprivation, any activities of daily living, impairment or immobility, vision impairment, hearing impairment or dehydration Exclusion Criteria: severe dementia (MMSE < 10), psychotic disorder; unable to consent or refused; terminal condition receiving comfort care; to be discharged within 48; any behavioral or medical condition that may place the volunteer's health and safety at risk Recruitment Method: patients able to communicate and aged greater than 70 years were enrolled on admission to the geriatric wards	N=37 Mean age (yrs): Intervention: 84 Control: 86 p=0.4 Gender, male (%): 22 Race/ethnicity (%): NR Medical unit: Geriatrics	Delirium incidence (CAM) Delirium severity (assessed using Memorial Delirium Assessment Score (MDAS)) Length of stay Cost analysis data provided	Allocation Concealment: NA Blinding: NR Intention to Treat Analysis (ITT): yes Withdrawals adequately described: none
Harari, 2007[66] United Kingdom Study Design: Prospective before-and-after study Funding Source(s): Guys and St. Thomas' Charity	Prevention Strategy Used: proactive care of older people undergoing surgery (POPS) – a multidisciplinary preoperative comprehensive geriatric assessment (CGA) and post-operative follow-up (n=54) Controls: pre-POPS (n=54)	Inclusion Criteria: elective orthopedic patients, age 65 and older Exclusion Criteria: none stated Recruitment Method: POPS targeted patients with risk factors for post-surgery complications; sought referrals for older patients needing surgery but considered too 'medically unfit"	N=108 Mean age (yrs): 74.6 Gender, male (%): 39.8 Race/ethnicity (%): NR Medical unit: elective orthopedic surgery	Delirium incidence (defined as acute change in mental status post-op with improvement pre-discharge) Length of stay Mortality (within 30 days)	Allocation Concealment: NA Blinding: outcomes assessment was non-blinded Intention to Treat Analysis (ITT): NA Withdrawals adequately described: all included

Author, Year, Country, Study Design, Funding Source	Prevention Strategy Used, Controls	Inclusion and Exclusion Criteria, Recruitment Method	Patient Characteristics (expressed in means unless otherwise noted)	Outcomes Evaluated	Study Quality
Naughton, 2005[67] United States Study Design: Cohort Funding Source(s): Non-industry (Kalieda Fdn & West NY AD Assistance Ctr)	Prevention Strategy Used: multifactorial: emergency physicians educated and reminded to evaluate patients >75 years old for dementia & delirium and to admit patients with dementia or delirium to the Acute Geriatric Unit (AGU); AGU protocol including nurse, physician and environmental interventions; nurse and physician education and feedback on performances (4-Month Outcome (n=154) and 9-Month Outcome (n=110)) Controls: pretest/ baseline patients admitted 9/98-11/98 to general med service (n=110)	Inclusion Criteria: ≥75 years, admitted to non-critical-care medical service of Buffalo General Hospital 4 months and 9 months after multi-factorial prevention program started Exclusion Criteria: admitted from nursing home, declined to be interviewed Recruitment Method: consecutive admissions to medical service	N=cohort of 110 patients evaluated at baseline (before prevention strategy implemented); cohort of154 patients evaluated 4 months after implementation; cohort of 110 patients evaluated 9 months after implementation; (total N=374) Mean age (yrs): baseline cohort: 81±6.2; 4-month cohort: 81±6.1; 9-month cohort: 82±5.9 Gender, male (%): baseline cohort: 41 (37%); 4-month cohort: 52 (34%); 9-month cohort: 38 (35%) Race/ethnicity (%): NR Medical unit: baseline cohort: general medicine; 4-month cohort: Acute Geriatric Unit (AGU; N=84) & general medicine (N=70); 9-month cohort: AGU (N=37) & general medicine (N=73)	Delirium prevalence (defined as +CAM) Medication use (benzodiazepines, antidepressants, antihistamines, opiates, neuroleptics)	Allocation Concealment: NA Blinding: NA Intention to Treat Analysis (ITT): NA Withdrawals adequately described: NA

Delirium: Screening, Prevention, and Diagnosis – A Systematic Review of the Evidence

Author, Year, Country, Study Design, Funding Source	Prevention Strategy Used, Controls	Inclusion and Exclusion Criteria, Recruitment Method	Patient Characteristics (expressed in means unless otherwise noted)	Outcomes Evaluated	Study Quality
Tabet, 2005[68] UK Study Design: single-blind case-control study Funding Source(s): NR	Prevention Strategy Used: intervention ward - educational package s delivered to medical and nursing staff, 3 components: (1) 1 hour session including a formal presentation and small group discussion; (2) written information and guidelines on how to prevent, recognize and manage delirium in older people; (3) regular one-to-one and small group discussions lasting up to an hour during which staff were encouraged to discuss discharged challenging cases they had encountered with the aim of enhancing their learning experience with specific examples (n=122) Controls: control ward -no educational package and established practice was maintained throughout (n=128)	Inclusion Criteria: 70 years of age or older, understood and spoke English, agreed to take part, had no recorded symptoms of delirium in medical and nursing notes on admission, and had been in hospital for longer than 24 hours Exclusion Criteria: NR Recruitment Method: all admissions to the two medical units between December 2001 and August 2002 were considered eligible for inclusion if they met the above criteria	N=250 Mean age (yrs): Intervention: 81 Control: 79 p=0.007 Gender, male (%): 48 Race/ethnicity (%): NR Medical unit: medicine	Point prevalence of delirium (defined using a modified Delirium Rating Scale (DRS))	Allocation Concealment: NA Blinding: single (patients) Intention to Treat Analysis (ITT): yes, however case notes of 6 patients on the intervention ward and 8 on the control ward could not be traced by the Medical Records Department and therefore were not examined Withdrawals adequately described: none reported
Wong Tim Niam, 2005[69] Australia Study Design: Before and after study Funding Source(s): NR	Prevention Strategy Used: program group - quality improvement methods including staff education and use of a checklist to facilitate use of the 10 strategies, including (1) maintenance of adequate brain oxygen delivery; (2) maintenance of fluid and electrolyte balance; (3) pain protocol; (4) active policy of discontinuing or minimizing medications; (5) regulation of bladder/ bowel function (6) adequate nutrition; (7) early mobilization and rehabilitation; (8) prevention, early detection and treatment of major peri- and post-operative complications; (9) appropriate environmental stimuli; (10) treatment protocol of agitated delirium (n=71) Control: no program group (n=28)	Inclusion Criteria: all patients with osteoporotic hip fracture aged over 50 years admitted during the study period Exclusion Criteria: < 50 years of age Recruitment Method: consecutive patients with hip fracture admitted to the orthopedic unit at Fremantle Hospital	N=99 Mean age (yrs): 82 Gender, male (%): 28 Race/ethnicity (%): NR Medical unit: orthopedic	Delirium incidence (assessed using CAM) Delirium duration Length of hospital stay	Allocation Concealment: NA Blinding: none Intention to Treat Analysis (ITT): yes Withdrawals adequately described: NA

Author, Year, Country, Study Design, Funding Source	Prevention Strategy Used, Controls	Inclusion and Exclusion Criteria, Recruitment Method	Patient Characteristics (expressed in means unless otherwise noted)	Outcomes Evaluated	Study Quality
Milisen, 2001[70] Belgium Study Design: Before and after study Funding Source(s): Government, Private Industry	Prevention Strategy Used: education of nursing staff; systematic cognitive screening; consultative services by delirium resource nurse, geriatric nurse specialist, or psychogeriatrician; scheduled pain protocol (n=60) Control:; usual care prior to implementation of intervention (n=60)	Inclusion Criteria: admitted to emergency department of one hospital with traumatic fracture of proximal femur and hospitalized in 1 of 2 traumatological nursing units within 24 hrs of surgery; Dutch speaking and verbally testable Exclusion Criteria: multiple trauma, concussion, pathological fractures, surgery occurring more than 72 hours after admission, aphasia, blindness, deafness, fewer than 9 years of formal education Recruitment Method: all patients approached by research nurses within 48 hours after admission	N=120 Median age (yrs): 81 Gender, male (%): 19 Race/ethnicity (%): NR Medical Unit: traumatological wards	Delirium incidence (based on CAM) Duration of delirium Mortality Length of stay	Allocation Concealment: NA Blinding: NA Intention to Treat Analysis (ITT): yes Withdrawals adequately described: NA

Delirium: Screening, Prevention, and Diagnosis – A Systematic Review of the Evidence

Author, Year, Country, Study Design, Funding Source	Prevention Strategy Used, Controls	Inclusion and Exclusion Criteria, Recruitment Method	Patient Characteristics (expressed in means unless otherwise noted)	Outcomes Evaluated	Study Quality
Inouye, 1999[71] Rizzo 2001[72] Inouye 2003[73] Leslie 2005[75] Leslie 2005[75] United States Study Design: controlled clinical trial Funding Source(s): National Institute on Aging and other local non-industry grants	Prevention Strategy Used: multi-component strategy (Elder Life Program); intervention consisted of standardized protocols for the management of six risk factors for delirium: cognitive impairment, sleep deprivation, immobility, visual impairment, hearing impairment, and dehydration (n=426) Controls: prospectively matched patients (n=426) Note: intervention strategy was implemented by a trained interdisciplinary team, which consisted of a geriatric nurse-specialist, two specially trained Elder Life specialists, a certified therapeutic-recreation specialist, a physical therapy consultant, a geriatrician, and trained volunteers	Inclusion Criteria: at least 70 years old, no delirium at the time of admission, and at intermediate or high risk for delirium at baseline Exclusion Criteria: inability to participate in interviews (because of profound dementia that precluded verbal communication, language barrier, profound aphasia, or intubation or respiratory isolation), coma or terminal illness, hospital stay of 48 hours or less, prior enrollment in this study Recruitment Method: all subjects in intervention unit who met the eligibility criteria were enrolled; concurrently, eligible patients from two usual-care units were identified, so subject pool was sufficiently large to permit use of a computerized algorithm designed to match patients according to age within five years, sex, and base-line risk of delirium (intermediate or high)	N=852 Mean age (yrs): 80 Gender, male (%): 39 Race/ethnicity (%): white 87 Medical unit: General medicine	Delirium incidence (defined according to the criteria of the CAM) Total days of delirium No. of episodes of delirium Delirium-severity score Recurrence (two or more episodes)	Allocation Concealment: Not feasible, but a prospective, individual matching strategy was chosen as an alternative to randomization Blinding: none stated Intention to Treat Analysis (ITT): yes Withdrawals adequately described: yes
Lundstrom, 1999[76] Sweden Study Design: prospective case series with 2 historical control case series (see Gustafson, 1991) Funding Source(s): several non-industry grants	Prevention Strategy Used: intervention program - staff education, co-operation between orthopedic surgeons and geriatricians, individual care and planning of rehabilitation, improved ward environment, active nutrition, improved continuity of care and prevention and treatment of complications associated with delirium (n=49) Controls: patients from two studies, one a control and one a medical intervention; all patients were 65 years of age and older consecutively admitted to an orthopedic hospital for femoral neck fracture repair (n=111 and n=103)	Inclusion Criteria: patients operated on for fractured neck of the femur Exclusion Criteria: NR Recruitment Method: patients with hip fractures from the study catchment area admitted to the department in which the orthopedic surgeon and the geriatricians co-operate in the treatment and care of the patients	N=49 (Intervention) Mean age (yrs): 79.7 Gender, male (%): 35 N=111 (Control 1) Mean age (yrs): 79.3 Gender, male (%): 25 N=103 (Control 2) Mean age (yrs): 79.5 Gender, male (%): 27 All Groups: Race/ethnicity (%): NR Medical unit: orthopedics	Diagnosed delirium (based on DSM-III-R criteria).	Allocation Concealment: NA Blinding: NR Intention to Treat Analysis (ITT): NA Withdrawals adequately described: NA

Author, Year, Country, Study Design, Funding Source	Prevention Strategy Used, Controls	Inclusion and Exclusion Criteria, Recruitment Method	Patient Characteristics (expressed in means unless otherwise noted)	Outcomes Evaluated	Study Quality
Wanich, 1992[77] United States Study Design: quasi-experimental Funding Source(s): foundation and government grants	Prevention Strategy Used: nursing staff education, subject orientation, communication with family, mobilization, environmental modifications, caregiver education, medication management, discharge planning (n=135) Controls: nursing care per unit staff (usual care) (n=110)	Inclusion Criteria: age 70 and older, admitted to study medical unit between Sunday noon and Friday noon Exclusion criteria: transferred from another unit within the hospital, admitted for short-stay procedure, admitted only for terminal care Recruitment Method: Consent sought within 24 hours of admission to study unit or control units	N=235 Mean age (yrs): 77 Gender, male (%): NR Race/ethnicity (%): NR Medical unit: non-critical care general medicine units with geriatric clinical specialist nurses in Intervention unit	Diagnosed delirium (based on Delirium Screening Assessment [MMSE#, BPRS#, and clinical exam] with psychiatrist making final diagnosis based on DSM-III) Hospital mortality Length of stay #MMSE=Mini-Mental State Examination BPRS=Brief Psychiatric Rating Scale	Allocation Concealment: NA Blinding: psychiatrist who made final diagnosis blinded to Delirium Screening Assessment Intention to Treat Analysis (ITT): NA Withdrawals adequately described: NA
Gustafson, 1991[78] Sweden Study Design: prospective case series with historical controls Funding Source(s): several foundation grants	Prevention Strategy Used: 1) surgical policy (operate as soon as possible), 2) pre-operative assessment and thrombosis prophylaxis 3) oxygen therapy, 4) anesthetic technique, and 5) post-operative assessment and treatments (n=103) Controls: patients seen in the same orthopedic department approximately 3 years prior to study period (n=111)	Inclusion Criteria: consecutive patients, 65 and older, fractured neck of the femur Exclusion criteria: none stated Recruitment Method: consecutive admissions	N=103 (Intervention) Mean age (yrs): 79.5 Gender, male (%): 27 N=111 (Controls) Mean age (yrs): 79.3 Gender, male (%): 25 Both Groups: Race/ethnicity (%): NR Medical unit: Orthopedic Surgery	Delirium incidence (acute confusion based in DSM-III criteria) Duration of delirium Orthopedic ward stay Mortality	Allocation Concealment: NA Blinding: NR Intention to Treat Analysis (ITT): NA Withdrawals adequately described: NA

83

Appendix D, Table 4. Primary Prevention Outcomes of Non-Pharmacologic or Mixed Studies

Author, Year	Delirium Incidence/ Prevalence n/N (%)		Delirium Severity		Delirium Duration, days (SD unless noted)		Length of Stay, days (SD unless noted)		Use of Rescue Medications n/N (%)	
	Intervention	Control	Intervention	Control	Intervention	Control	Intervention	Control	Intervention	Control
Randomized trials										
Lundstrom, 2007[55] *Specialized geriatric ward, multi-disciplinary education and multi-component intervention*	56/102 (54.9) p<0.01 Delirium ≥ 1 during hosp. after day 7 18/102 (18.4) p<0.001 Delirious on day of discharge 0/102 p<0.001	73/97 (75.3) Delirium ≥ 1 during hosp. after day 7 50/97 (51.5) Delirious on day of discharge 20/97 (20.6)			5.0 (7.1) p=0.01	10.2 (13.3)	28.0 (17.9) p=0.03 Delirious pts. only 31.4 (19.3) p=0.03	38.0 (40.6) Delirious pts. only 43.6 (42.7)	Sedatives (delirious pts.) 6/39 (15.4) p<0.01 Opioids (delirious pts.) 12/39 (30.8) p<0.01	Sedatives (delirious pts.) 20/48 (41.7) Opioids (delirious pts.) 29/47 (61.7)
Taguchi, 2007[56] *Bright light*	1/6 (16.7) p=0.42	2/5 (40.0)								
McCaffrey, 2006[57] *Music*	2/62 (3.2) p<0.01	36/62 (58.1)								
Lundstrom, 2005[58] *Staff education & multi-component intervention*	63/200 (31.5) p=0.91 Remain delirious on day 7 19/63 (30.2) p<0.01	62/200 (31.0) Remain delirious on day 7 37/62 (59.7) p<0.01					9.4 (8.2) p<0.001	13.4 (12.3)		
Marcantonio, 2001[59] *Proactive geriatrics consultation*	20/62 (32) p=0.04 Severe delirium 7/62 (12) p=0.02 Delirium at discharge 8/62 (13)	32/64 (50) Severe delirium 18/64 (29) Delirium at discharge 12/64 (19)			2.9 (2.0) (per episode) p=NS	3.1 (2.3) (per episode)	5 (2) (median and IQR) p=NS	5 (2) (median and IQR)		

Author, Year	Delirium Incidence/ Prevalence n/N (%)		Delirium Severity		Delirium Duration, days (SD unless noted)		Length of Stay, days (SD unless noted)		Use of Rescue Medications n/N (%)	
	Intervention	Control	Intervention	Control	Intervention	Control	Intervention	Control	Intervention	Control
Non-randomized studies										
Ushida, 2009[60] *Decreased steroids and immediate post-surgical movement with cervical orthosis*	3/38 (7.9) p=0.01	23/81 (28.4)								
Vidan, 2009[61] *Multi-disciplinary education & multi-component intervention*	20/170 (11.7) p<0.05	69/372 (18.5)	Based on CAM, range 0-7 4.9 (0.4) p=0.08	Based on CAM, range 0-7 5.3 (1.0)	*Hours* 31.1 (43.0) p=0.73	*Hours* 33.6 (22.0)				
Kratz, 2008[62] *Education & multi-component nursing intervention*	Protocol units (4.7)	Control units (11.0)								
Robinson, 2008;[63] Vollmer 2007[64] *Nursing and nursing assistant education and multi-component intervention*	Protocol 11/80 (13.8) p<0.001	Pre-protocol 30/80 (37.5)								

Delirium: Screening, Prevention, and Diagnosis – A Systematic Review of the Evidence

Author, Year	Delirium Incidence/ Prevalence n/N (%)		Delirium Severity		Delirium Duration, days (SD unless noted)		Length of Stay, days (SD unless noted)		Use of Rescue Medications n/N (%)	
	Intervention	Control	Intervention	Control	Intervention	Control	Intervention	Control	Intervention	Control
Caplan, 2007[65] *Multi-component intervention via volunteers and nursing assistants*	1/16 (6.3) p=0.03	8/21 (38.1)	Based on MDAS (scale not provided) 1.2 p<0.05	Based on MDAS (scale not provided) 5.1	5 (only 1 subject, no SD) p=0.64	12.5 (14.5)	22.5 (9.6) p=0.35	26.8 (17.8)		
Harari, 2007[66] *Pre-op geriatric assessment and post-op follow-through*	Protocol 3/54 (5.6) p=0.04	Pre-Protocol 10/54 (18.5)					11.5 (5.2) p=0.03	15.8 (13.2)		
Naughton, 2005[67] *ER and geriatric unit physician and nurse education & multi-component intervention*	4-month cohort: 35/154 (22.7); p<0.01 9-month cohort: 21/110 (19.1); p<0.001	Baseline 45/110 (40.9)					*Non-delirious pts only* 4- and 9 month cohorts combined (n=208) 8.2	*Delirious pts only* Baseline (n=45) 11.5	*Significant differences from baseline* 4-mo cohort: Anti-depressants: 29/154 (19%); p<0.05 9-mo cohort: Benzo-diazepines: 11/110 (10%); p<0.01 Anti-histamines: 4/110 (4%); p<0.01 Opiates: 25/110 (23%); p<0.01	Benzo-diazepines: 34/110 (31%) Anti-depressants: 11/110 (10%) Anti-histamines: 17/110 (16%) Opiates: 47/110 (43%) Neuroleptics: 12/110 (11%)
Tabet, 2005[68] *Staff education*	12/122 (9.8) p=0.03	25/128 (19.5)								
Wong Tim Niam, 2005[69] *Multi-component intervention recommended by geriatric registrars*	Post-intervention 9/71 (12.7) p=0.01	Baseline period 10/28 (35.7)			Baseline period 5 (2-6) p=0.43	Post-intervention Median (range) 3 (2-4)	Baseline period Median (range) 8 (3-41); p=NS	Post-intervention Median (range) 10 (2-44)		

Author, Year	Delirium Incidence/ Prevalence n/N (%)		Delirium Severity		Delirium Duration, days (SD unless noted)		Length of Stay, days (SD unless noted)		Use of Rescue Medications n/N (%)	
	Intervention	Control	Intervention	Control	Intervention	Control	Intervention	Control	Intervention	Control
Milisen, 2001[70] *Inter-disciplinary education and multi-component intervention*	12/60 (20.0) p=NS	14/60 (23.3)	Post-op Day 1: 2.73 Day 3: 3.82 Day 5: 3.36 Day 8: 1.91 (Total CAM score), p=0.02	Post-op Day 1: 6.92 Day 3: 5.78 Day 5: 6.54 Day 8: 6.0 (Total CAM score)	1 (1) (median and IQR) p=0.03	4 (5.5) (median and IQR)	13 (6.5) (median and IQR) p=NS	16 (5.25) (median and IQR)		
Inouye 1999,[71] Rizzo 2001,[72] Inouye 2003,[73] Leslie 2005[75] Leslie 2005[74] *Inter-disciplinary multi-component intervention*	Episodes 62 p=0.03 First episode 42/426 (9.9) p=0.02	90 First episode 64/426 (15.0)	‡3.85±1.27; p=0.25	3.52±1.44	Total days 105 p=0.02	161	Median 7 days	Median 7 days		
Lundstrom, 1999[76] *Inter-disciplinary education and multi-component intervention*	Post-op 15/49 (30.6) p<0.001 vs. Control 1 (C1); p<0.05 vs. Control 2 (C2) Delirium ≥ 7 days 8/49 (16.3) p<0.01 vs. C1, p=0.09 vs. C2	Post-op C1 68/111 (61.3) C2 49/103 (47.6) Delirium ≥ 7 days Control 1 44/111 (39.6) Control 2 29/103 (29.1)					Ward (ortho-pedic) stay 12.5; p=NR	Ward (ortho-pedic) stay C1 17.4 C2 11.6		
Wanich, 1992[77] *Inter-disciplinary education and multi-component intervention*	26/135 (19.0) p=0.61	22/100 (22.0)								
Gustafson, 1991[78] *Multi-component intervention*	Post-op 49/103 (47.6) p<0.05 Severe 7103 (6.8) p<0.0001 More than 7 days 30/103 (29.1)	Post-op 68/111 (61.3) Severe 33/111 (29.7) More than 7 days 44/111 (39.6)					Orthopedic Ward 12.8 (10.4) p<0.01	Orthopedic Ward 20.0 (15.4)		

Appendix D, Table 5: Characteristics of Intensive Care Unit Diagnostic Accuracy Studies

Author, Year Country Funding	Level of Evidence	Inclusion and Exclusion Criteria Recruitment Method	Patient Characteristics	Index Test(s) and Examiner Reference Standard and Examiner	Outcomes Evaluated
Bergeron, 2001[114] CANADA Funding: NR	2	Inclusion: admitted to medical and surgical ICU for >24 hours Exclusion: diagnosis of delirium on admission, comatose or stuporous	N= 93 Mean age (yrs): 62 Gender, male (%): 52 VETERAN (Y/N): N Race/ethnicity (%): NR Medical unit: med/surg ICU Comorbid conditions (list): NR APACHE II 14 (8–21)	ICDSC – ICU physician Diagnosis by consulting board certified psychiatrist	Validation of ICDSC
McNicoll, 2005[115] USA Funding: government, foundation	2	Inclusion: consecutive patients admitted to ICU, ≥65 years Exclusion: no appropriate surrogate, transferred from another ICU, non-English speaking, inability to communicate, intubated, mechanically ventilated, or physically restrained	N= 22 Mean age (yrs): 78 Gender, male (%): 36 VETERAN (Y/N): N Race/ethnicity (%): caucasian 73 Medical unit: ICU Comorbid conditions (list): visual/hearing impairments (38%), history of alcohol use (33%), disability in ADLs (37%), preexisting cognitive impairment (45%) APACHE 25.9 CHARLSON 2.0	CAM-ICU - trained clinician researchers CAM - trained clinician researchers	Sensitivity and specificity of CAM and CAM-ICU
van Rompaey, 2007[120] Belgium Funding: NR	5	Inclusion: non intubated, score of at least 10 on Glasgow Coma Scale, 18 years or older; ICU stay of at least 24 hours before first assessment Exclusion: none stated	N= 172 Mean age (yrs): 60 Gender, male (%): 59 VETERAN (Y/N): N Race/ethnicity (%): NR Medical unit: ICU Comorbid conditions (list): NR APACHE II: 21	NEECHAM – trained nurse researcher CAM-ICU - same nurse researcher	Comparison of NEECHAM with CAM-ICU Length of stay
Hart, 1996[109] USA Funding: institutional grant	4	Inclusion: patients with delirium (from ICU), schizophrenia (inpatient), or depressive illness(inpatient) (all by DSM-III-R criteria) or dementia (outpatient) Exclusion: history of substance abuse, major medical illness, or neurologic disorders	N= 103 (22 with delirium) For Delirium Patients: Mean age (yrs): 62.5 Gender, male (%): 54.5 VETERAN (Y/N): N Race/ethnicity (%): African American 50, caucasian 50 Medical unit: ICU Comorbid conditions (list): NR APACHE: NR	CTD – bachelor's level psychologist technician DSM III-R-psychiatrist	How well CTD performed across 4 populations (delirium, dementia, depression, schizophrenia)

Author, Year Country Funding	Level of Evidence	Inclusion and Exclusion Criteria Recruitment Method	Patient Characteristics	Index Test(s) and Examiner Reference Standard and Examiner	Outcomes Evaluated
Ely, 2001[110] USA Funding: government, foundation	3	Inclusion: admitted to ICU Exclusion: history of severe dementia, psychosis or neurologic disease; patient or family refusal; comatose	N= 38 Mean age (yrs): 60 Gender, male (%): 60 VETERAN (Y/N): N Race/ethnicity (%): caucasian 84, African American 14, Hispanic 2 Medical unit: ICU Comorbid conditions* (list): acute respiratory distress 29%, MI or arrhythmia 16%, CHF 16%, hepatic or renal failure 13%, COPD 11%, GI bleeding 8%, malignancy 5% APAHCE II: 17.1	CAM-ICU – study nurses and intensivists DSM IV – geriatrician, geriatric consult-liaison psychiatrist	Validation of CAM-ICU
Pisani, 2006[111] USA Funding: foundation	3	Inclusion: medical ICU patients, 60 years and older Exclusion: no proxy, patient died during proxy interview, transfer from other ICU; in ICU<24h, non-English speaking	N= 178 Mean age (yrs): 74.2 Gender, male (%): 52 VETERAN (Y/N): N Race/ethnicity (%): non-caucasian 12 Medical unit: ICU Comorbid conditions (list): dementia (29%), disability in ADLs (31%), GI hemorrhage* (16%), respiratory* (51%), neurologic* (2%), sepsis* (17%) APACHE II: 23.4 CHARLSON: 1.9	Chart-based delirium method – trained research nurse CAM-ICU—trained research nurses	Validation of chart-based delirium detection method
Ely, 2001[116] USA Funding: government, foundation	2	Inclusion: medical and coronary ICU patients, mechanically ventilated Exclusion: history of psychosis and neurologic disease, inability to communicate (non-English speaking, deaf, comatose), extubated before assessment, previously enrolled in the study, refusal to participate	N= 96 Mean age (yrs): 55.3 Gender, male (%): 47.9 VETERAN (Y/N): N Race/ethnicity (%): caucasian 79.2, black 19.8, Hispanic 1.0 Medical unit: ICU Comorbid conditions* (list): acute respiratory distress 35%, cancer 15%, myocardial infarction or arrhythmia 9%, hepatic or renal failure 9%, CHF 6%, COPD 6%, GI bleeding 5%, drug overdose 3%, other 12% APACHE II: 22.9	CAM-ICU – critical care study nurses DSM IV – geriatrician delirium expert, board certified geriatric consult-liaison psychiatrist, or neuropsychologist	Validation of CAM-ICU Length of stay
Spronk, 2009[121] Netherlands Funding: NR	5	Inclusion: ICU stay >48 hours Exclusion: preexisting neurocognitive dysfunction, documented dementia, language barriers or deafness, active psychiatric disorder, severe neurologic disorder	N= 46 Mean age (yrs): 73 Gender, male (%): 65 VETERAN (Y/N): N Race/ethnicity (%): NR Medical unit: ICU Comorbid conditions (list): NR APACHE II: 18	Clinical judgment – ICU nurses and physicians CAM-ICU - research nurses	Validation of clinical judgment Length of stay Mortality

89

Author, Year Country Funding	Level of Evidence	Inclusion and Exclusion Criteria Recruitment Method	Patient Characteristics	Index Test(s) and Examiner Reference Standard and Examiner	Outcomes Evaluated
van Eijk, 2009[122] Netherlands Funding: NR	1	Inclusion: all (adult) admissions to ICU (medical 24%, surgical 25%, cardiothoracic surgical 29%, neurological/neurosurgical 22%) Exclusion: deeply sedated, comatose, deaf, did not speak Dutch or English, did not consent	N= 126 Mean age (yrs): 62.4 Gender, male (%): 72 VETERAN (Y/N): N Race/ethnicity (%): NR Medical unit: ICU Comorbid conditions (list): NR APACHE II: 20.9	CAM ICU – trained ICU study nurses ICDSC – patient's bedside ICU nurse Diagnostic impression –critical care intensivist, fellow, or resident DSM IV - psychiatrist, neurologist, geriatrician	Validation of CAM-ICU, ICDSC, and physician impression
Guenther, 2010[123] Germany Funding: government, industry	2	Inclusion: all admissions to ICU Exclusion: coma, acute stroke, refusal, non-Germanspeaking	N= 54 Mean age (yrs): 67 Gender, male (%): 69 VETERAN (Y/N): N Race/ethnicity (%): NR Medical unit: ICU Comorbid conditions* (list): Abdominal surgery 13%, vascular surgery 6%, urology 2%, lung surgery 1%, cardiac surgery 23%, trauma 4%, ear/nose/throat surgery 2% APACHE: NR	CAM-ICU Flowsheet – intensivist, trained medical student DSM IV - psychiatrist	Validation of CAM-ICU Flowsheet
Plaschke, 2008[117] Germany Funding: foundation	5	Inclusion: admitted to ICU after elective surgery or after emergency, age 18 or older Exclusion: profound hearing or vision impairment, non-German speaking, coma or unconscious	N= 174 Mean age (yrs): 62.4 Gender, male (%): 70.1 VETERAN (Y/N): N Race/ethnicity (%): NR Medical unit: ICU Comorbid conditions* (list): pancreas resection 32%, GI 21%, cardiorespiratory 19%, urology/renal failure 10%, metabolic disease 9%, polytrauma 4%, other 5% APACHE II: 25 p/m	ICDSC - trained nurses CAM-ICU - physician researcher NOTE: study compared agreement of these 2 tools	Agreement of the ICDSC and CAM-ICU Length of stay Mortality
Shyamsundar, 2009[118] India Funding: NR	5	Inclusion: admitted to medical or cardiac ICU, age 13 or older Exclusion: unable to speak, intubated, refused consent	N= 120 Mean age (yrs): 54.9 Gender, male (%): 72.5 VETERAN (Y/N): N Race/ethnicity (%): NR Medical unit: ICU Comorbid conditions (list): NR APACHE: NR	MDAS – junior resident ICD-10 (International Classification of Diseases, 10th revision) – psychiatrist (unclear if all patients were evaluated by psychiatrist)	Validation of MDAS Interrater reliability

Author, Year Country Funding	Level of Evidence	Inclusion and Exclusion Criteria Recruitment Method	Patient Characteristics	Index Test(s) and Examiner Reference Standard and Examiner	Outcomes Evaluated
Koolhoven, 1996[119] UK Funding: NR	5	Inclusion: admitted after elective cardiac surgery, >21 years of age Exclusion: refused, death	N= 15 Mean age (yrs): 63 Gender, male (%): 80 VETERAN (Y/N): N Race/ethnicity (%): NR Medical unit: ICU Comorbid conditions (list): NR APACHE: NR	Observation checklist (based on DRS) - study physicians DSM III R - unclear	
Lin, 2004[113] China Funding: government	1	Inclusion: in ICU, mechanically ventilated Exclusion: history of dementia, psychosis, mental retardation, other neurologic disease; receiving antipsychotics or high dose morphine or midazolam; under general anesthesia or heavily sedated, refused	N= 102 Mean age (yrs): 73.4 Gender, male (%): 53 VETERAN (Y/N): N Race/ethnicity (%): NR Medical unit: ICU Comorbid conditions* (list): pneumonia (31%), lung disease (24%), stroke (11%), cancer (8%), CHF (5%), GI disease (5%), diabetes or metabolic disorder (5%), myocardial infarction (3%), drug intoxication (3%) APACHE III: 64.9	CAM-ICU - 2 research assistants DSM IV - psychiatrists	Validation of CAM-ICU Mortality Interrater reliability
Luetz, 2010[112] Germany Funding: NR	1	Inclusion: newly admitted to ICU after surgery, age ≥ 60, LOS at least 24h Exclusion: preexisting psychosis, dementia, depression, non-German speaking, inability to communicate	N= 156 Mean age (yrs): 69.8 Gender, male (%): 55 VETERAN (Y/N): N Race/ethnicity (%): NR Medical unit: ICU Comorbid conditions* (list): general surgery (39%), cardiac (25%), trauma (16%), gynecologic (9), urologic (4%), otorhinolaryngological (4%), vascular (2%), oral (1%) APACHE II: 18	CAM-ICU, Nu-DESC, DDS – trained physicians and nurses DSM IV – board-certified psychiatrist or intensivist	Validation of CAM-ICU, Nu-DESC, and DDS Interrater reliability Length of stay Discharge disposition

*ICU admission diagnosis

APACHE = Acute Physiology and Chronic Health Evaluation; NR = not reported; ADLs = Activities of Daily Living;
CAM-ICU = Confusion Assessment Method – Intensive Care Unit; CAM = Confusion Assessment Method; CTD = Cognitive Test for Delirium; DDS = Delirium Detection Score; DSM = Diagnostic and Statistical Manual of Mental Disorders; ICDSC = Intensive Care Delirium Screening Checklist; MDAS = Memorial Delirium Assessment Scale; NEECHAM = Neelon and Champagne Confusion Scale; Nu-DESC: Nursing Delirium Screening Scale